Horse and Pony Ailments

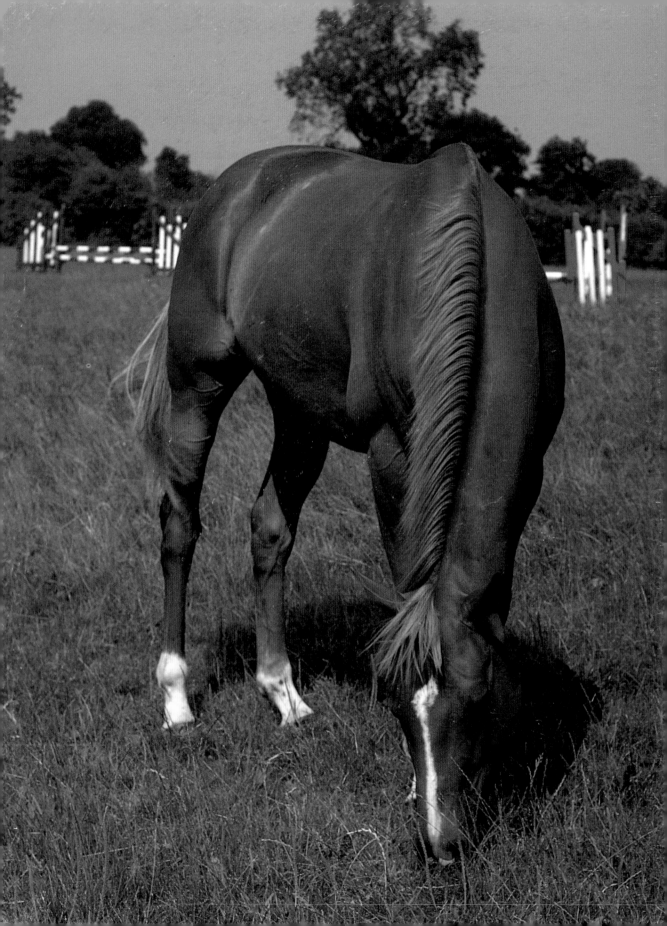

Horse and Pony Ailments

Eddie Straiton

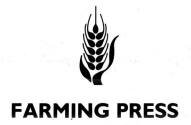

FARMING PRESS

First published 1971
as *The TV Vet Horse Book: recognition and treatment
of common horse and pony ailments*

Ninth edition 1992
retitled as *Horse and Pony Ailments*

ISBN 0 85236 213 7

A catalogue record for this book is available
from the British Library

**Published by Farming Press Books
Wharfedale Road, Ipswich IP1 4LG, United Kingdom**

Distributed in North America
by Diamond Farm Enterprises,
Box 537, Alexandria Bay, NY 13607, USA

Cover design by Mark Beesley
Phototypeset by Typestylers Ltd, Ipswich
Printed and bound in Great Britain
by Butler & Tanner Ltd, Frome and London

We acknowledge with thanks permission to reproduce the horse's stomach
(page 38) and larynx (page 94) from *The Anatomy of the Domestic Animal*
by Sisson and Grossman, 4th ed, published by W.B. Saunders Company.
We also thank The Cooper Technical Bureau for permission to reproduce
the mange illustration on page 43.

Contents

To John Harvest

Preface to the Ninth Edition

When I entered the veterinary profession I recognised the need for an easily understood horse reference book and I always meant to produce one just as soon as I could write with absolute authority. Although in 1971 my experience was considerable I thought that such a book would have to wait a few years. Then a golden opportunity presented itself. Harry Robb, who had taught me as a student at Glasgow Veterinary College, retired and settled down just over thirty miles from my hospital. Harry had all the necessary qualifications — a long lifetime in practice crammed with intensive horse work. In fact few, if any, living veterinary surgeons could match his equine experience. I had found the ideal consultant literally on my doorstep.

In order to produce the initial manuscript I travelled the sixty-odd miles to and from Harry's farm twice weekly for several months. Harry taped his memories of each condition and we transcribed and discussed the tapes together, often grilling each other late into the night. Subsequently I photographed all the cases in my practice and the first edition of this book, published in 1971, was the result.

In each succeeding edition the language has been kept simple so that it can be understood by even the youngest of owners and riders. At the same time it has always been designed to be equally valuable to adult horse owners, to veterinary students and to successive generations of veterinary surgeons with limited horse experience.

Each updated edition has continued to emphasise basic commonsense advice, much of which has survived throughout the last two hundred years. The number of photographs has grown steadily, and this is the first edition with colour photographs integrated throughout the text.

On completing the original manuscript I learned with great sadness of the passing of Harry Robb. It is my wish therefore that the book should be a permanent and sincere memorial to his name. He was without doubt one of the finest veterinary surgeons and gentlemen I have ever had the privilege of knowing.

I acknowledge the skill of my photographer Tony Boydon, who is responsible for the majority of the pictures, and also the courtesy of the horse owners who cooperated in the photography.

Eddie Straiton
1992

Horse and Pony Ailments

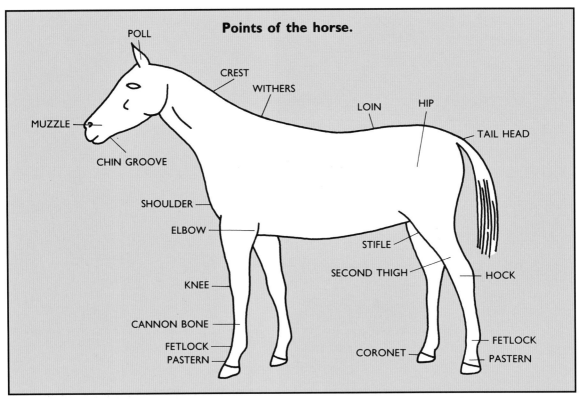

Points of the horse.

POLL
CREST
WITHERS
MUZZLE
CHIN GROOVE
LOIN
HIP
TAIL HEAD
SHOULDER
ELBOW
STIFLE
SECOND THIGH
HOCK
KNEE
CANNON BONE
FETLOCK
PASTERN
CORONET
FETLOCK
PASTERN

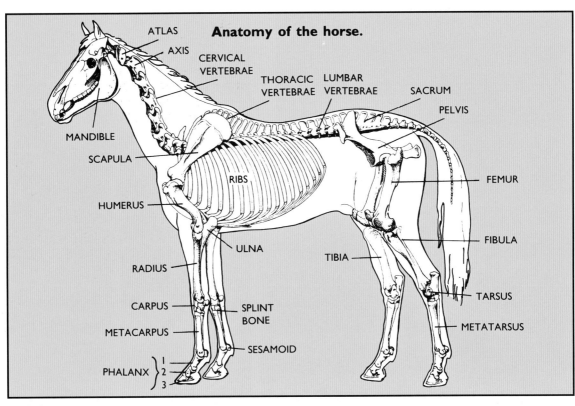

Anatomy of the horse.

ATLAS
AXIS
CERVICAL VERTEBRAE
THORACIC VERTEBRAE
LUMBAR VERTEBRAE
SACRUM
PELVIS
MANDIBLE
SCAPULA
RIBS
FEMUR
HUMERUS
ULNA
FIBULA
RADIUS
TIBIA
CARPUS
SPLINT BONE
TARSUS
METACARPUS
METATARSUS
SESAMOID
PHALANX 1 2 3

Introduction

NORMALITY IN THE HORSE

Normal body temperature 100.4 – 100.8°F
(38 – 38.2°C)
Normal pulse   35 – 45 per minute
Normal respirations   8 – 12 per minute

As a general rule the larger the horse, the slower the pulse. For example, the pulse in a Shire averages 35 per minute, whereas in the Shetland pony the average is nearer 45.

By the same token respirations in the Shire average 8 per minute and in the Shetland 12.

The body temperature varies with age, being slightly higher in younger animals.

FIRST-AID KIT

The mistake made by most horse owners is to stock up with an excessive quantity and variation of first-aid remedies, with the result that when there is an emergency they waste valuable time wondering which to use.

The ideal is to keep a comparatively small box (*photo 1*) containing the following:

1. About 8 oz of a bland antiseptic. If in any doubt about which to choose, get your veterinary surgeon to supply it

2. One small packet of surgical gauze, preferably in a roll

3. A 1 lb roll of cotton wool

4. Half a dozen surgical bandages — ideally 3-4 inches width, as anything smaller is impractical

5. Four oz of sulphonamide (this can be supplied only by your veterinary surgeon)

Suggested routine
A wound is most frequently on the legs. Having cleaned up and dressed it with sulphonamide, cover with gauze. Pass a layer of cotton wool over the gauze and completely round the leg. Hold in position with a bandage (*photo 2*), and then ring for your veterinary

2

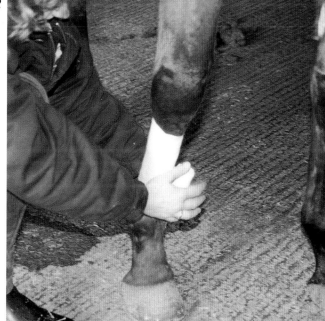

1

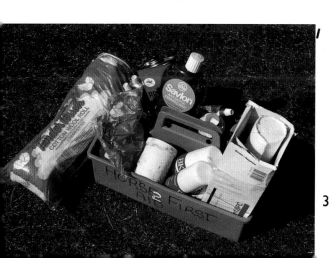

3

surgeon. Use the gauze under the wool to prevent strands of the wool adhering to the wound.

After your veterinary surgeon has inspected and treated the wound, he will no doubt tell you to leave the bandages off as soon as possible since wounds heal more quickly when exposed to the atmosphere. He will also most likely inject the patient with tetanus antitoxin to provide immediate protection.

1
Breeding

A simple knowledge of breeding is invaluable to all horse owners. There is little doubt that more and more people are going in for horse breeding, especially in the pony world. Often, when a child outgrows the pony, the question arises as to what to do. The pony can be sold, but frequently it has become part of the family and no-one wants to sell it. If it is a mare, then the obvious thing to do is to breed from her (*photo 1*).

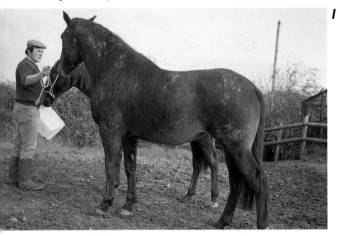

1

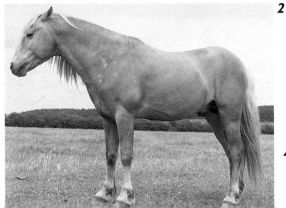

2

The first question — which stallion or sire should be used? Naturally one should pick a stallion of good conformation and movement, but the most important thing of all is temperament (*photo 2*). One should never use a stallion with a bad temperament; this major fault is nearly always hereditary. A bad natured pony is not only a nuisance but can be a real danger to the handlers as well as the child.

Having selected the sire, the next question that arises is — when should the mating take place? In thoroughbreds that are going to be used for racing it is desirable to have the foal born as early in the year as possible. This is because, in thoroughbreds, the foal ages from the 1st of January in each year and, if it is being raced as a two-year-old on the flat, then the extra one or two months are always an advantage.

With ponies, hacks and hunters, however, this does not arise and it is better to have the foals born when the weather is good and there is plenty of grass, i.e. in May or towards the end of June, depending on whether in the South or North of the country.

The period of gestation, i.e. the time the foal is carried (between service of mare and birth of foal), is approximately eleven months, though on odd occasions it may be a week or two shorter or up to a month longer. Therefore, if the foal is to be born in May, the service should be given in June.

The mare will come into season every three weeks and will stay in season and willing to take the stallion for two to three days. During this time, within the mare, the female egg, i.e. the ovum, is shed from the ovary. For conception to take place the ovum has to unite with the spermatozoa from the stallion.

The spermatozoa live only for approximately 24 hours; if they do not meet the egg or ovum during that time the service will be a failure.

The ideal time to have the mare mated is towards the end of her heat period. This provides a maximum chance that the ovum has been shed. It is a good idea, and certainly a practical one, to consult your veterinary surgeon at this stage. He may decide to examine the mare *per rectum* (*photo 3*), and to rupture the follicles or egg-containers in the ovaries to make sure that the egg is shed before service.

Forty to sixty days after service it is a good idea to get your veterinary surgeon to take a blood sample from the mare and have it checked for pregnancy. A urine sample can be tested three to four months after service.

While the mare is in-foal she must be well cared for and well fed. This is vital in procuring a strong healthy foal.

When a mare is going to foal
As foaling time approaches, the udder or vessel of the mare will commence to swell. A waxiness develops on the teats (*photo 4*), and they may start to run milk. However, despite these general signs, it is very difficult to tell exactly when a mare is going to foal. She doesn't like being watched during her foaling and will often get on with it during the night. In fact I have known many people who have sat up night after night, week after week, without witnessing the birth. They have then either fallen asleep or gone for a cup of coffee, and the foal has been there when they next looked.

When the mare does start to foal, the process is very rapid and, if everything is normal, will be all over in 15 to 30 minutes.

Foaling inside or at grass
This is a matter of personal preference and there is no definite rule.

After the foal is born, the placenta or afterbirth — a large red or chocolate coloured

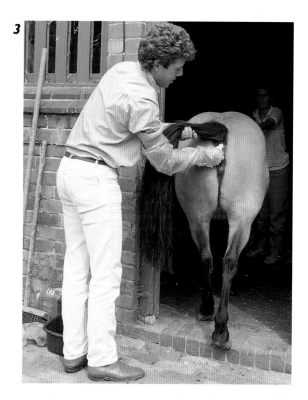

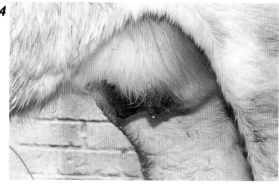

membrane in which the foal has been enclosed — must be passed by the mare (*photo 5*). If

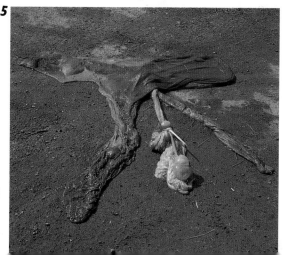

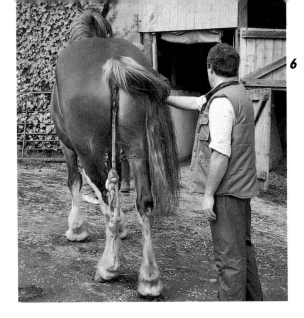

this has not happened within two hours, then the veterinary surgeon must be summoned immediately. If the afterbirth is left inside the mare, very serious and often fatal conditions can arise such as metritis, laminitis, pneumonia and septicaemia (*photo 6*).

Handling the foal
When the foal is two or three days old, a small head collar should be fitted (*photo 7*). The foal can then be led around following the mother. This ought to be done every day; if it is, then

6 the foal will soon settle down to handling and this will save a great deal of trouble later. The simple rule to follow is to get the foal leading at the earliest possible moment and keep it leading.

Early handling also allows detailed identification of the foal.

Weaning
The foal should be weaned, i.e. taken away from its mother, in the autumn. From then on it will be able to feed and take care of itself, but even then it should still be handled and led about every day. It is a good idea to handle the legs and lift the feet frequently and this, like the leading, should be started as early as possible. This leg handling and foot lifting will be tremendously beneficial in the future, both to the handlers and the blacksmith.

Castration
If the foal is a colt, he will have to be castrated, unless, of course, he is a valuable breeding animal. This is usually done at one year old, but in certain parts of the country it is now common practice to perform the operation earlier. Needless to say, this operation must be done by a veterinary surgeon. (See chapter on 'Castration'.)

When should the youngster be worked?
Whether the youngster is a colt or a filly, it cannot be put into hard work — showing, jumping or hunting — until it is four years old.

Four years is a long time to wait, and if the youngster is a filly, then it is practical and economical to put her to the stallion and let her breed a foal during this time. If the filly is mated as a two-year-old (*photo 8*), then she

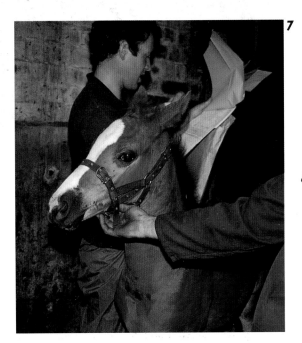

7

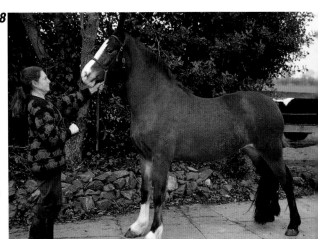

8

will foal as a three-year-old and will be ready to go into hard work as a four-year-old. Not only is this a vital economy hint, but foaling at three years old will make the filly drop her belly and look much better.

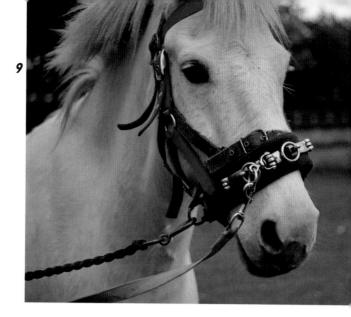

Treatment before four years old

As a two-year-old, after service the filly can be mouthed, driven in long reins, girthed and even backed. After the foal is born, the mouthing, girthing, backing, etc. can be carried on with the foal by the mare's side in the field.

A special lungeing head collar (*photo 9*) will make the initial work much easier.

The same treatment should be meted out to the colt from two years onwards.

At four years old both the colt and the filly are ready for any job.

Best time to serve after foaling

With a brood mare kept entirely for breeding, the best time for service is as soon as she comes in season after the foal is born. This is usually around ten days after birth and is the ideal time to re-mate the brood mare for the production of a foal the following year. The younger the mare the better the chance she has of holding to this service.

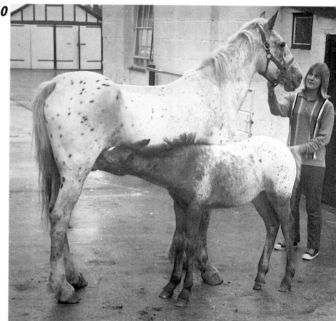

When is a mare too old to breed?

A mare is never too old to breed whether or not she has bred before, though obviously it is much better if she starts her breeding career at an early age. The pelvis in the young animal is more cartilaginous and relaxes easier. Nonetheless, early service is not vital or essential. The mare with foal in photo 10 was 24 years old at the time.

2
Foaling

When the foal is in the uterus (i.e. the womb), it requires blood and oxygen to keep it alive and growing. This is supplied by the mother, through the placenta and via the umbilical cord.

The umbilical cord contains three tubes, viz. the umbilical artery, the umbilical vein and the urachus.

The umbilical artery carries fresh oxygenated blood from the mother. This oxygenated blood passes to the foal's heart and is then pumped throughout the body. Since the foal is not breathing, the blood bypasses the lungs. It returns via the umbilical vein to be re-oxygenated in the mother's lungs.

The urachus is connected with the foal's bladder and carries away the urine into one of the two watery sacks which surround the foal and cushion it against damage.

When the mare starts to foal, her uterus contracts producing the so-called 'labour pains'. The contractions force the watery sacs against the cervix, or entrance of the womb, causing the cervix, to open up. The continued labour then forces the sacs down the vagina (almost like a very soft hydraulic ram) and these open up the passage to make ample room for the foal to pass out.

If you are lucky enough to watch a foal being born, the first thing you will see appearing at the lips of the vulva will be what looks like a large balloon full of liquid. This will rupture and copious quantities of fluid will rush out, to be followed almost immediately by the fore feet and the nose of the foal.

By the time this stage is reached, the mare's labour pains and strains are tremendously powerful and the rest of the foal soon appears. If it doesn't, then a veterinary surgeon should be called immediately.

The majority of mares lie down when foaling, but occasionally a mare will deliver the foal whilst standing. Do not interfere — both are natural positions.

After the birth

When the foal is completely out, it will generally be still attached to the mother by the umbilical cord. **Do not rush to rupture or cut this**. Nature provides that the blood should drain from the placenta and umbilical cord into the foal. After a certain length of time the mare will stand up, or the foal will start to struggle, and the cord will stretch and rupture as nature intended it to.

Some people ligature the umbilical cord and then cut it. I prefer to let it rupture naturally, though it is a wise precaution to dress the part of the cord left attached to the foal with one of the modern antibiotics to prevent the entrance of infection.

The foal should be on its feet and sucking within an hour (*photo 1*). When the foal attempts to get up, it will half rise and fall over on several occasions: it is better *not* to assist the foal to rise. The energy expenditure is good for the foal and each attempt strengthens it. Let it get up on its own and then guide it, if you like (though this should not be necessary), towards the mare's udder and check that it is sucking. That this is not necessary is evidenced by the simple fact that foals born outside with no-one in attendance rarely look back.

If you find the mare stretched out, straining heavily and making no progress, with nothing or perhaps just one leg showing, then send for your veterinary surgeon immediately (*photo 2*).

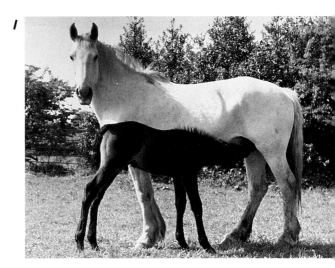

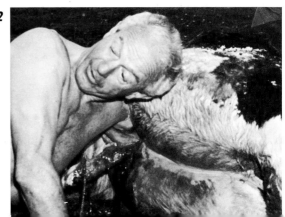

8

Sometimes after foaling, haemorrhage may occur from surface vaginal vessels. This can be rectified by cauterisation or cryosurgery (*photo 3*).

Milk substitute for rearing the foal
If the mare has insufficient milk, it may be necessary to supplement the foal's feed. For this purpose I have found the most satisfactory mixture to be:

3½ pints of cow's milk
½ pint of lime water (mix a handful of lime in a bucket of water and let the lime settle)
2 tablespoonfuls of glucose
6 drops of cod-liver oil

Cow's milk with 2 tablespoonfuls of glucose or sugar added is also satisfactory.

Your veterinary surgeon can feed the foal by stomach tube if it won't suck the substitute from a bottle.

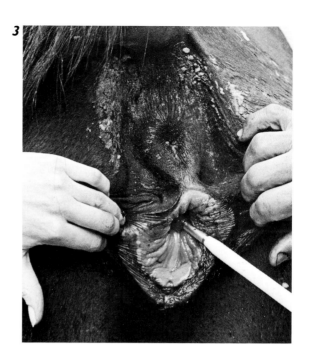

3
Equine Metritis

A venereal disease of brood mares which first appeared in Britain in 1977.

Cause
A gram negative coccobacillus with many similarities to the gonococcus of man.

Mode of spread
The infection is apparently spread from affected to clean mares by the stallion but there is some evidence that it may also pass between in-contact mares.

Symptoms
Failure to hold to service with or without a profuse mucopurulent discharge, which appears within 48 hours of the mare being covered (*photo 1*).

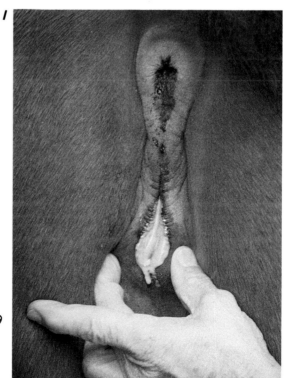

N.B. Any mare may show a discharge (purulent or otherwise) 24-48 hours after service due to local vaginal damage and/or infection.

The vast majority of such mares have sufficient natural immunity to resolve this in three or four days without interfering with a pregnancy.

Treatment
The mare
Intra-uterine infusion of broad-spectrum antibiotics daily for three to five days. This can be combined with intramuscular injections of the same antibiotic.

The stallion
A scrupulous cleansing of the sheath and penis using a special chlorhexadine solution, followed by a daily dressing for five days with a nitrofurazone cream or ointment.

Prevention
Routine veterinary examination of a cervical and vaginal smear taken from the mare, combined with the use of a known clean stallion.

The possibilities of a vaccine are being explored by scientists, but personally I think the disease will eventually be controlled by the extended use of artificial insemination.

4
Haemolytic Disease

A disease of the new-born foal seen mainly from the mare's fourth pregnancy onwards.

Cause
After several foalings the colostrum or first milk from the mare may contain antibodies which clash with those in the red blood corpuscles of the foal. Such foal antibodies are acquired from the stallion. The clash between the respective antibodies triggers off a haemolytic anaemia in the foal.

Symptoms
The foal appears perfectly normal and healthy at birth. From eight hours onwards is the vulnerable time. Foals under three days old are usually severely affected and die within 24 to 36 hours, showing progressive lethargy, weakness, anaemia and, after 24 hours, jaundice. The heart sounds become increasingly audible.

Older foals show milder symptoms and often recover without treatment.

Treatment
If the foal is over five days of age the only treatment required is a quiet, warm, dry loose box. Any excitement can jeopardise the foal's life. With young foals treatment is very much a job for your veterinary surgeon.

Prevention
Where the possibility of this disease is suspected the danger can be confirmed by blood testing the mare late in pregnancy.

In such cases the foal has to be muzzled at birth and fed every four hours for the first 24-36 hours with milk substitute. At the same time the mare's udder should be stripped out also at four-hour intervals.

Colostrum from another mare, if obtainable, should be given to the foal during this period as should also long-acting antibiotic and perhaps blood serum from another mare.

Obviously with all such suspect mares it is best to send them to specialised quarters at foaling time.

5
Other Problems in the Foal

Constipation

In the foal's intestine there is firm dark chocolate-brown or almost black faeces (dung). This is known as the meconium and it is essential that it passes out as quickly as possible. During the first two or three days the mare's milk (the colostrum) contains a substance called cholestron; this is a laxative designed by nature to make the bowels work and get rid of the meconium.

If within six to eight hours this meconium has not been passed, it is wise to assist it by giving a liquid paraffin enema (*photo 1*). Four ounces of liquid paraffin may be given by the mouth, but the enema is quicker and more certain. This is a job for your veterinary surgeon since, if the meconium is not passed, the foal stops sucking, develops colicy pains and may even die.

Diarrhoea

During the first 48 hours of life the foal may develop acute diarrhoea. This is generally due to excess cholestron in the milk.

The treatment is to take the foal away for 24 to 48 hours and hand-milk the mare (*photo 2*). Put the foal onto a bottle of cow's milk, with sugar added to it, every four hours right through the 24 hours.

If the foal is valuable it is wise to have the milk given, by the veterinary surgeon, through a stomach tube (*photo 3*). The foal will

2

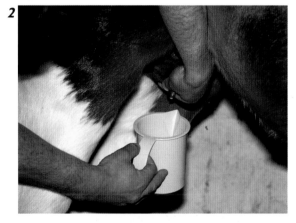

1

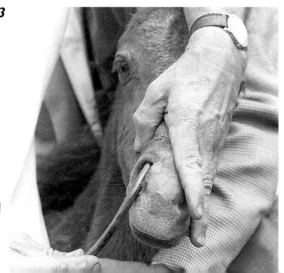

3

improve rapidly as soon as the cholestron is cut off.

Infectious diarrhoea — bacterial scour

Later, diarrhoea may occur again. If it does, it is nearly always due to a bowel infection, perhaps secondary to the original dietetical upset.

Such cases require expert veterinary attention immediately because bacterial scour in the foal is a very serious condition.

Usually the veterinary surgeon will leave the foal on the mare but will give antibiotic injections along with antibiotics and kaolin by the mouth (*photo 4*). The kaolin — a white powder — is best given mixed with boiled milk since this stops the foal taking too much fresh milk from the mother.

With either of these conditions, the foal may go downhill rapidly and look critically ill but, like all young animals, when the cause is removed the recovery is just as spectacular. Laboratory examination of the faeces will show the specific organisms involved.

Pervious urachus

This occurs when the urachus — the tube which has taken the urine away during pregnancy — fails to wither up after the foal is born and urine drops continuously from the navel.

Treatment is surgical and is usually successful. Your veterinary surgeon should be called in as soon as possible because there is always a risk that infection will travel up the urachus and set up a cystitis (i.e. inflammation of the bladder).

Joint-ill or navel-ill

This is a pyogenic disease of foals, i.e. it is caused by bacteria that form pus.

The bacteria gain entry into the foal via the navel or through scratches or cuts on the body. They travel via the blood to the joints, where they start to multiply producing, heat, pain, swelling (*photo 5*), and, if not treated quickly, pus.

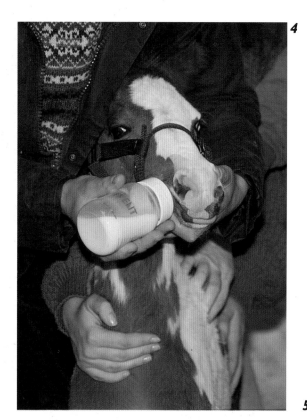

4

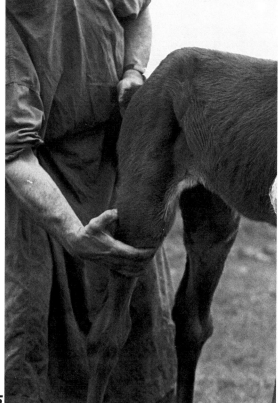

5

Symptoms

The first sign is lameness in one or more legs (*photo 6*). Any lameness, no matter how slight, in the foal should be regarded as a suspect joint-ill and should be reported to your veterinary surgeon immediately.

If untreated, one or more joints start to swell and are exceedingly painful. The pulse and temperature are both elevated with the temperature up to 105° or 106°F (40.5° or 41°C). Needless to say, the foal stops sucking and has great difficulty in rising, standing or lying down.

6

Treatment

Successful treatment depends on immediate action so get in touch with your veterinary surgeon as soon as possible. He will inject specific and broad-spectrum antibiotics (*photo 7*), and may reinforce his treatment with oral sulpha drugs. Results can be, and

often are, spectacular, but remember the treatment must be started before the pus forms.

Prevention

Dress the navel after birth with a reliable antibiotic or sulpha drug, both of which can be supplied by your veterinary surgeon.

Vaccines can be tried but they are variable in their results and should never be totally relied on. Good husbandry — cleanliness in the foaling box if foaled inside, etc. — plus the conscientious dressing of the navel probably give as good if not better protection than do the vaccines.

A long-acting (seven day) penicillin injection given at birth and repeated in five days provides an excellent insurance but only when combined with good husbandry.

Simultaneous with the first dose the foal should be injected with tetanus antitoxin which gives a ten-week protection.

7

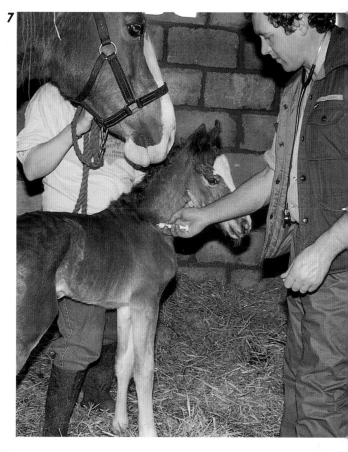

13

6
Rickets

Rickets, occasionally known as metabolic bone disease, can develop in any horse up to three years of age though mostly it affects foals; and though the signs can start to show early on, they usually appear in foals between six months and one year old (*photo 1*).

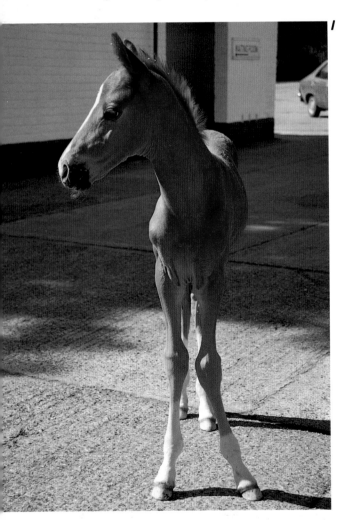

1

It is a disease of the ends of the long bones rather than of the joints, though the distorted bone ends produce ragged joint surfaces, which naturally predispose to arthritis if the condition is not correctly treated quickly.

Cause

Rickets arises from what we call metabolic upsets, i.e. functional disturbances in the liver, which can be described as the 'factory of the body' where the simple products of intestinal digestion are elaborated and built up before being transported to various parts of the anatomy to provide heat and energy, minerals and vitamins to build up and replace bone, muscle, brain, etc. Rickets occurs when there is a deficiency of any one mineral or vitamin or an imbalance in the combination of the minerals calcium and phosphorus, and the vitamins D, C or A.

Vitamin A and carotene (vitamin C) are vital for the correct metabolism or utilisation of calcium and phosphorus. Plenty of phosphorus is required to ensure the proper absorption of vitamins A and C. Sunshine helps to produce natural vitamin D.

Treatment

Careful dieting under veterinary supervision combined with vitamin and mineral injections. Also sunshine and moderate exercise.

The most effective surgical treatment is illustrated in photos 2-7. The foal is first anaesthetised (*photos 2 & 3*) and then the operation site is prepared (*photo 4*). The incision is made (*photo 5*), and a staple is inserted at the side of the joint (*photos 5 & 6*). An X-ray shows that the staple is in the correct position (*photo 7*).

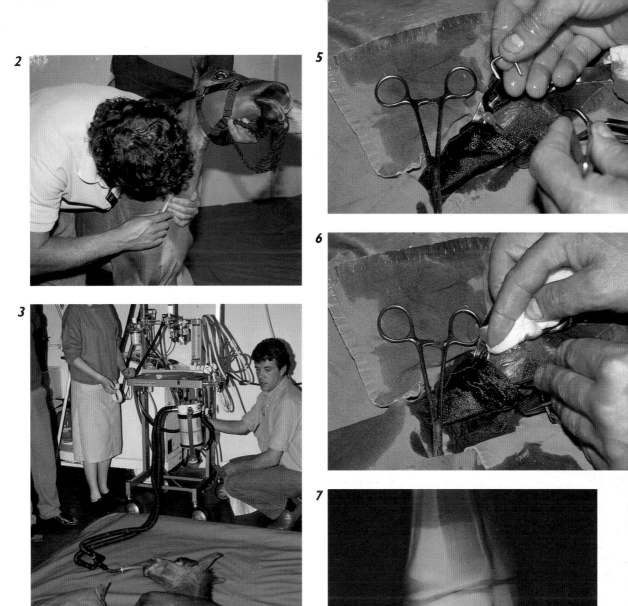

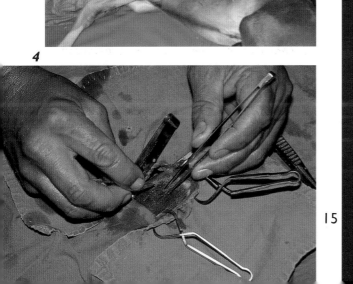

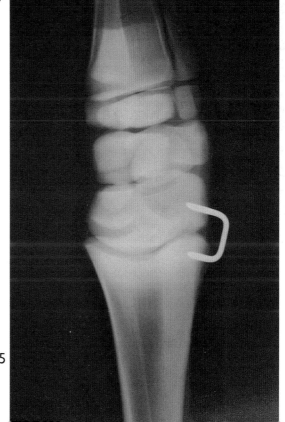

15

Prevention

Make sure the mare's rations, and those of the foal when it starts to eat, contain reasonable amounts of all the components mentioned above.

If there is a deficiency of vitamin A, the horses' coats will be rough and dull. Rations high in protein mainly of grain often contain practically no vitamin A.

If you see either mare or foal chewing at fences, tree bark or any other wood, then you've probably got a deficiency of calcium or phosphorus, though the same wood chewing can occur when vitamins C and D are in short supply.

A substance called phytic acid found in oats can also interfere with the metabolism of calcium.

Good hay (and remember only the best is good enough for horses) should provide all the calcium and phosphorus needed, but in addition I advise moderate quantities (2-4 lb) of compound nuts with an added vitamin supplement together with a fairly liberal daily helping of chopped carrots (to provide the vitamin C).

Bran is rich in phosphorus so a small mash daily is indicated (2-4 lb).

7
Hernias

Occasionally a foal is born with an umbilical hernia (*photo 1*) or a small hernia in the inguinal region. In such cases wait until the foal is a yearling and then get your veterinary surgeon to operate.

If the hernia is large with any danger of bowel strangulation, the operation may be performed just as soon as the foal can stand an anaesthetic.

The technique is illustrated in photos 2-5. Check that any bowel in the swelling is returned to the abdomen (*photo 2*). Insert two sharp sterile needles, in the form of a cross, through the base of the hernia sac; then

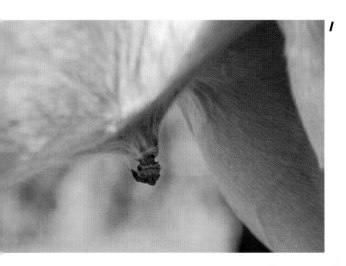

2

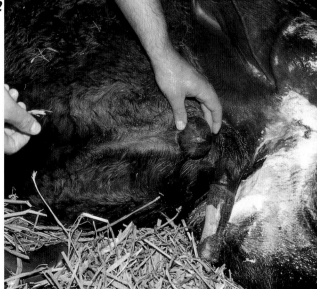

1

fit several elastic rubber rings over the needles and around the hernia as close to the abdomen as possible (*photo 3*).

Bind elastoplast round the hernia sac (incorporating the sharp ends of the needles to anchor it). Then cut off the sharp ends and bend back the stumps (*photo 4*).

Inject the patient against tetanus and against any possible infection. The ligated sac eventually drops off leaving perfect healing (*photo 5*).

See also 'The Ruptured Colt' in Chapter 8.

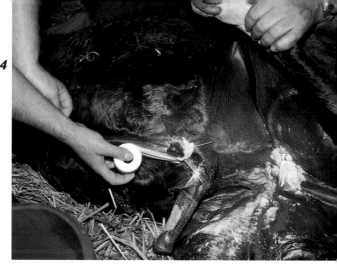

4

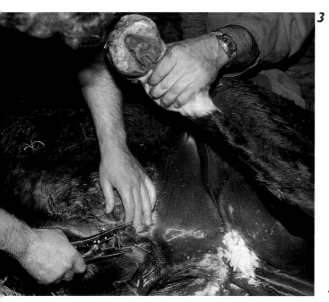

3

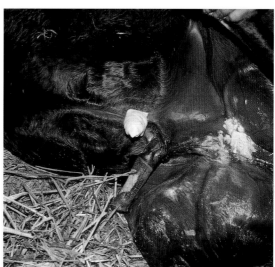

5

8
Castration

Opinion varies widely on the best age to castrate. Some veterinary surgeons now castrate foals.

There is no doubt that the retention of the testicles, at least for a time, helps the male horse to develop in conformation and temperament, so perhaps the best way of deciding when to have the operation performed is to wait until the young stallion becomes a 'nuisance'. He may then be a yearling, a two-year-old or even a three-year-old.

Tools for the job
The operation will be performed by your veterinary surgeon, but it will add interest to

the keeping of your gelding to understand something of the technique involved.

From my own experience, standing castration is preferable. Approximately one hour before commencing I inject a heavy dose of the tranquilliser acetylpromazine. Then I use an ecraseur (*photo 1*) — a chain on a ratchet to crush the spermatic cord thereby preventing fatal haemorrhage.

Method of restraint

For standing castration all that is required is a twitch or a twitch plus blinkers. Blinkers can be improvised by using a sweater or a towel (*photo 2*). Needless to say, a sensible assistant, who is not afraid of horses, is required to hold the head.

Injection against tetanus

Always, before starting any operation, the patient is given an injection of tetanus antitoxin. This is vitally important in all equine surgery.

The anaesthetic

In addition to the sedative or tranquilliser, a local anaesthetic is injected into each testicle and into the corresponding scrotum. The twitch and blinkers are then removed and the patient is left for quarter to half an hour to allow the anaesthetic to freeze completely the area and the spermatic cord.

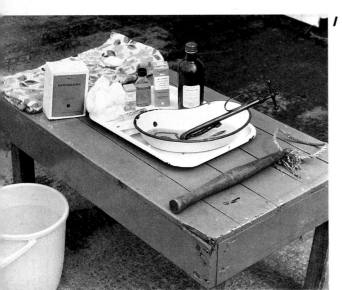

2

The operation

The testicles are exposed in turn, using a bold incision with an ultra sharp scalpel, and the cords are crushed through one by one with the ecraseur chain. The wounds are then dressed with sulphanilamide powder.

Clean cutting

The colt is cut clean when the epididymis — the small white bulb indicated here (*photo 3*)

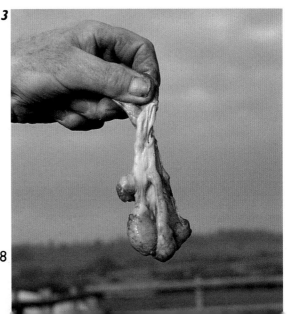

1

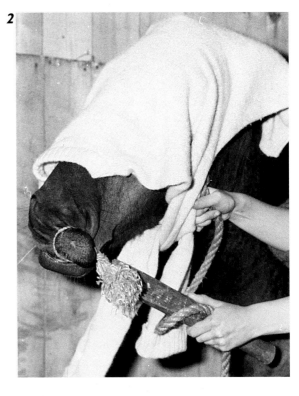

3

— is completely removed. When a stallion is 'cut proud' the epididymides are left inside; this is often done on circus horses. The small portion of testicular tissue left gives them a boldness and a carriage which geldings often lack.

No after-care should be necessary. Swelling of the area is inevitable (*photo 4*), but so long as the patient keeps eating there is no cause for concern. If he should go off his food, then send for your veterinary surgeon immediately.

If a permanent hard lump remains, then a chronic staphylococcal infection is the most likely cause. This condition called scirrhous cord should be reported at once to your veterinary surgeon. He will administer a general anaesthetic and will dissect out the infected portion of the spermatic cord.

Alternative to standing castration

For the less experienced veterinary surgeon the drugs Immobilon and Revivon offer a most acceptable alternative to the standing technique.

Immobilon is given intravenously and puts the horse down within seconds (*photo 5*). I also use a local anaesthetic as with the standing method.

The advantages are that skilled assistance is not so necessary, and with the colt down, it is easier to make sure that the crushing takes place well above the epididymis. An emasulator is the instrument most commonly used (*photo 6*).

After the operation Revivon (½ cc per cwt) is given intravenously, along with a single ½ cc subcutaneously, and within a very short time the patient is back on his legs (*photo 7*).

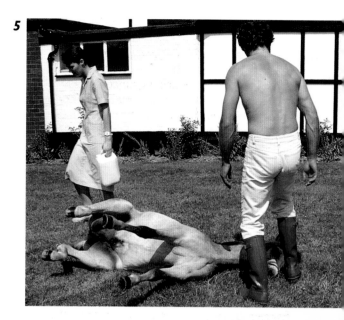

5

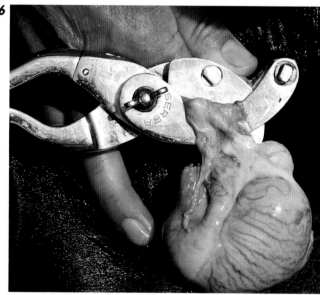

6

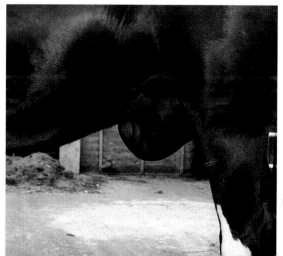

4

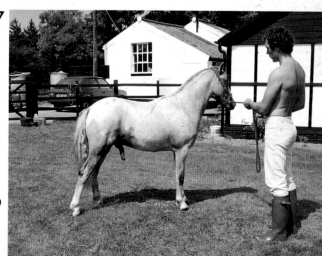

7

19

When using this technique I ligate the spermatic cord and its peritoneal covering well above where I apply the emasculator. This is an insurance against possible bowel prolapse.

THE RUPTURED COLT

Occasionally a colt is presented for castration with a scrotal hernia, i.e. a rupture causing the bowel to descend into the scrotum or sac in which the testicle is contained (*photo 8*).

Such a case requires specialist surgery under deep general anaesthesia. The tunica vaginalis (a fold of peritoneum which immediately surrounds the testicle) is blunt-dissected as high as possible back into the inguinal canal. The tunica-covered testicle is held firmly in one hand and during the dissection the descending bowel is replaced in the abdomen.

The tunica vaginalis, which now contains only the spermatic cord, is twisted twice and a clamp (*photo 9*) is applied tightly. This clamp is left to drop off on its own, which it usually does within three weeks.

The operation is normally a success and can be embarked on with complete confidence.

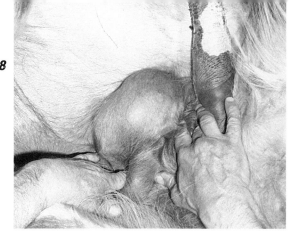

8

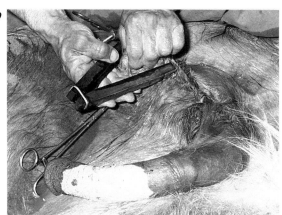

9

9
The Rig

A rig is a male horse which has retained one testicle in its abdomen or in its inguinal canal — the channel that runs from the scrotum to the inside of the abdomen.

Symptoms
A rig behaves like a stallion and is a real nuisance, especially when mares are present. He is difficult to handle and often difficult to ride.

Diagnosis and treatment
This is very much a matter for your veterinary

surgeon. He will take a blood sample from the suspect rig, then inject intravenously a large dose of luteinising hormone (usually about 6,000 IU) (*photo 1*). Half an hour later he will take a second blood sample and label it accordingly. He will then send both samples to one of the veterinary universities where the laboratory staff will examine them (especially the second one) for the male hormone testosterone. If none is present, the patient is not a rig.

If testosterone can be identified, then the veterinary surgeon will cast the animal and

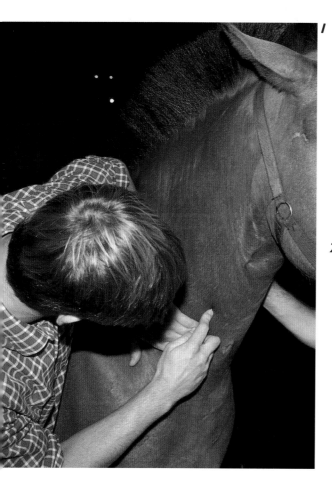

examine the scrotum for castration scars. One scar only will confirm that one testicle only has been removed. He will then explore the inguinal canal on the side opposite to the scar.

If the missing testicle cannot be felt, he will have to open into the abdomen through the flank and search for the testicle among the animal's intestines. A mid-line site is also used. In fact I now prefer it.

The operation is usually a complete success and will always justify the expense.

Sometimes the abdominal testicle is cystic or has atrophied, i.e. wasted way (*photo 2*).

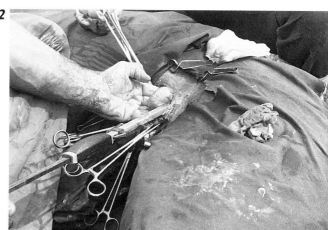

10
The Nymphomaniac

Nymphomania occurs in mares and is caused by cyst formation in one or both ovaries.

Symptoms
A mare with cystic ovaries can be even more difficult to handle and ride than a rig. In bad cases the mare is constantly in season and may kick or bite for no apparent reason.

Mild cases are manifest by general nappiness and when this persists in a mare a veterinary surgeon should be called in to examine the ovaries. In fact any fractious mare should be suspect.

Treatment
The only satisfactory treatment is the surgical removal of the ovaries. The operation is not easy but is usually highly successful.

After three days of dietetical preparation, deep closed circuit anaesthesia is induced and the mare's hindquarters are rolled on to thick sawdust-filled cushions.

Using a concealed knife and a special ecraseur chain on a long handle (*photo 1*), the offending ovaries are removed one by one from the vagina (*photo 2*).

No after-treatment is required.

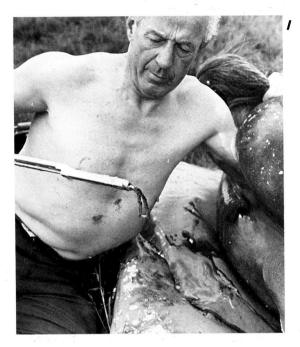

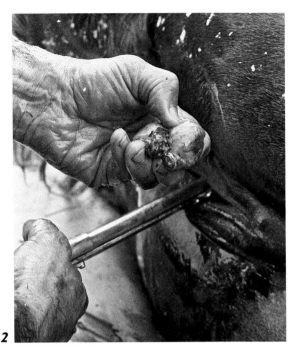

11
Simple Methods of Restraint

Horses and ponies are not unlike children — they like their own way and usually misbehave if they are allowed to get away with it. This can be an embarrassing nuisance, especially if you have to examine, clip, or treat them.

There are four simple methods of restraint which, used singly or together, usually allow the satisfactory handling of any horse.

Lifting a front foot
Obviously, standing on three legs, the horse is less likely to kick or prance about (*photo 1*).

Holding the tail
This is a specially useful hint during the examination of a hind leg. The horse will rarely kick if the tail is held firmly downwards, upwards, or to one side (*photo 2*).

Blindfolding
In my experience this is one of the most valuable of all the methods of restraint, especially if the animal has to be handled in an open field. Any first-aid blindfold can be used such as blinkers (*photo 3*) or a towel, a sweater, a coat or a sack.

Blindfolding is also useful when loading a nervous animal into a horse box or trailer.

A horse will rarely — if ever — kick when he cannot see.

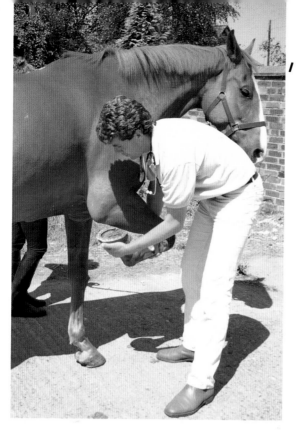

1 Applying a twitch

As a rule, this is only necessary when slight pain, such as a hypodermic injection, has to be administered, or if the horse hasn't been handled much. The muzzle is particularly sensitive and the pressure here distracts attention from the interference elsewhere. A combination of blinkers and the twitch (*photo 4*) will usually allow the satisfactory handling of even the most fractious of colts.

The twitch can also be applied around the base of an ear, where it works equally well, though this method should be resorted to only when all else fails because of the danger of permanent ear damage.

Needless to say, the horse should always be approached from the near (left) side.

Apart from these simple methods of restraint, common sense is of the greatest value. For example, if possible the owner or regular handler should always fit the halter, head collar or bridle and hold the head. Also when approaching from the near (left) side and during the entire examination, speak quietly to keep the horse informed of your whereabouts.

The majority of horses, even the untrained ones, respond best to a gentle approach and unhurried movements.

Never be afraid or excited; if or when you are, the horse will sense your emotions and will play up accordingly.

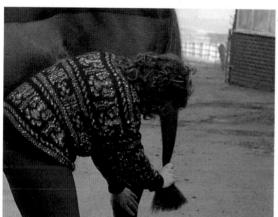

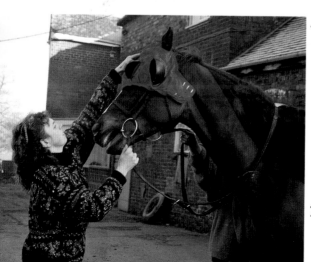

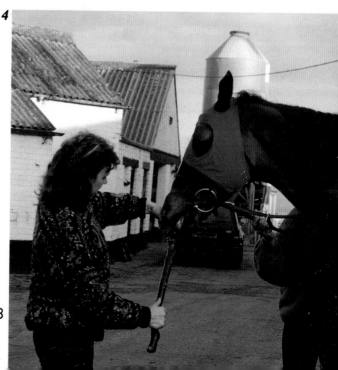

12
Wounds

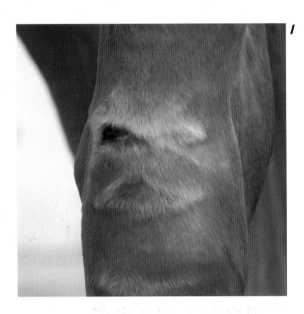

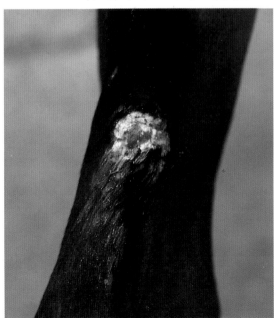

1 There are three types of wounds: incised wounds (i.e. cuts), tears, punctured wounds.

The incised wounds are those made either by the surgeon's knife or by sharp tin or sharp glass.

A typical tear wound is that caused by barbed wire (*photo 1*).

Punctures are caused by stakes or thorns or by a picked-up nail (*photo 2*).

In incised wounds the blood vessels — either arteries or veins or both — are cut clean through and the resulting haemorrhage is very severe.

In tears, the vessels are pulled and extended and there is practically no haemorrhage. This is because the walls of the veins and arteries are elastic, and when pulled, the ends recoil within themselves and form a natural barrier.

The same usually holds good for punctured wounds, though if the puncture is directly through a large vessel the resultant haemmorrhage can be fatal.

2

Treatment

Incised wounds

1. Control the haemorrage.
2. Clean the wound thoroughly and apply a sulphonamide or antibiotic dressing.
3. Get your veterinary surgeon to stitch the wound (*photo 3*). He will no doubt reinforce the dressing and inject against tetanus.

Tears

1. Control the haemorrhage.
2. Clean and dress the wound.
3. Get the wound stitched and the horse immunised against tetanus. However, if the wound is in a good position for drainage and healing (*photo 4*), stitching is not necessary.

24

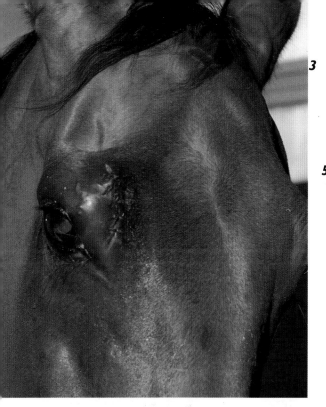

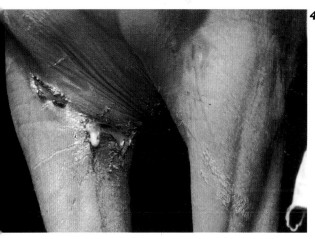

3 Cleaning the wound
This should be done thoroughly with warm water containing a bland or non-irritant antiseptic (*photo 5*); cotton wool or a clean cloth will help to remove any surface contamination.

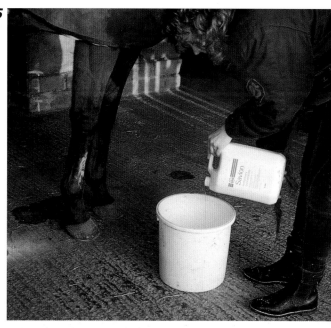

One very important point — never use iodine or any of the other old fashioned irritant antiseptics; all of these damage the tissues and retard healing. There are many non-irritant antiseptics on the market, most or all of which will destroy the bacteria without damaging the tissues.

The modern highly efficient dressings are the sulphonamides and the antibiotics, which will be prescribed by your veterinary surgeon.

To repeat, perhaps the most vital thing of all: ***Never forget that in the horse the great danger with any wound is tetanus.*** Antitoxin or antiserum should always be injected immediately, no matter how much toxoid the horse may have had during the previous year or years.

THE GRANULATING WOUND

When extensive wounds are healing, particularly tears, proud flesh very often forms

Punctures
1. Control the haemorrhage.
2. Dress with sulphonamide or antibiotic.
3. Ask the veterinary surgeon to inject against tetanus. Even though the horse may be immunised, the veterinary surgeon will give a booster protective dose of tetanus antitoxin. Remember, punctured wounds are the most dangerous of all, so far as tetanus is concerned. The veterinary surgeon will not suture a punctured wound unless a large blood vessel is directly involved.

(*photo 6*). When this happens, the wound is described as a granulating wound. If such granulations are not controlled by correct treatment, full union will be delayed for many months.

Treatment

As soon as the granulations appear, the wound should be dressed daily with a mild caustic solution. I have found the ideal dressing in such cases to be the same lotion recommended for the treatment of grease; that is, zinc sulphate ½ oz, lead acetate ¼ oz, water 1½ pints. If the granulations are excessive it may be necessary to keep the area covered with cotton wool soaked in the lotion, renewing the dressing daily, at least until the wound surface is level with the adjacent skin.

Where the granulation is excessive and chronic (*photo 7*) the only answer is 'pinch grafting' which requires the skills of an experienced veterinary surgeon. He will cut the growth off to slightly below the skin level and implant over the whole area minute pieces of skin taken from the horse's flank.

BROKEN KNEES

Broken knees occur when a horse or pony stumbles and falls on the road or on hard ground.

Cause

Fatigue, perhaps after a hard day's hunting or after an arduous ride when the horse is not in full working condition.

Long toes, seen when the shoes are left on too long or when the animal is badly shod, can also cause stumbling — as can excess weight on the pony's back.

Repeated stumbling can be associated with blood circulatory problems, so any persistent stumbler should be examined by a veterinary surgeon.

Symptoms

I think the term 'broken knees' describes the condition perfectly (*photo 8*). The wounds are usually lacerated and completely unsuitable for stitching. Fortunately the capsule of the knee

6

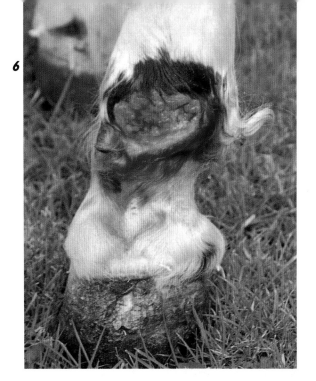

7

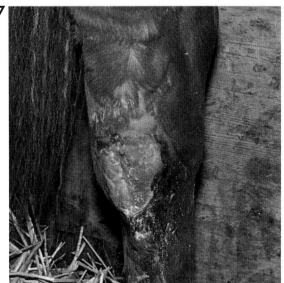

8

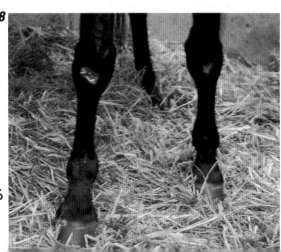

26

joint is very tough and is only rarely ruptured. If it is, then yellow synovial fluid will be seen in the discharge.

Occasionally if the horse falls on a stone or a sharp object a loose flap of skin may cover the wound.

If yellow synovial fluid (the so-called joint-ill) is seen coming from the wound, then prompt skilled veterinary attention is absolutely vital.

Treatment

An immediate injection of tetanus anti-toxin is essential in all cases of broken knees because of the danger of tetanus spores having been forced into the wound by the weight of the fall.

The wounds should be cleaned thoroughly with soap-flakes and warm water containing a non-irritant antiseptic and dried with a clean towel. They should then be dusted over with a sulpha powder twice or three times daily (*photo 9*). If the wound is extensive and

gaping, it is probably better to bandage with gauze, cotton wool and elastoplast after applying the sulpha powder. If there is a flap of skin, it will be necessary to get the veterinary surgeon to cut it off (*photo 10*).

As soon as the granulation tissue or proud flesh reaches the skin level, the daily dressing should be changed to the mild caustic lotion of zinc sulphate and lead acetate used for a granulating wound.

The wounds take a considerable time to heal, but the vast majority of broken knees recover completely.

Prevention

Correct feeding according to the work done and regular monthly shoeing keeping the toes as short as possible. Make certain that the horse or pony is well up to your weight.

10

9

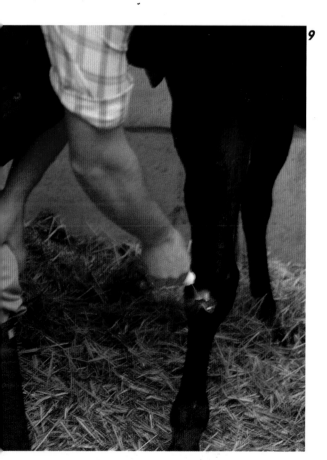

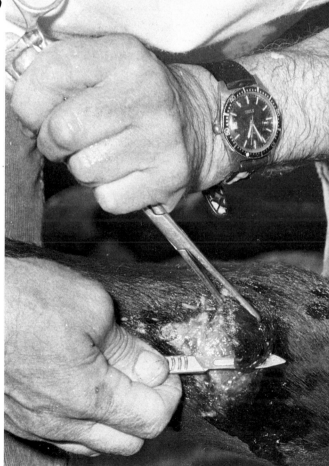

13
Haemorrhage

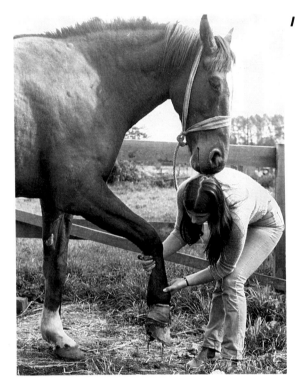

1 The word haemorrhage means simply bleeding (*photo 1*). There are two types:

    1. Venous, from a vein or veins.

    2. Arterial, from an artery or arteries.

Obviously the arterial bleeding is more dangerous than that from the veins, and it is important to be able to distinguish between the two.

In venous bleeding the blood 'oozes' or 'flows' (*photo 2*). In arterial bleeding the blood 'spurts out' in conjunction with the heart beats which are forcing the blood through the arteries.

Treatment

In general, bleeding is controlled by simple pressure.

Horses' legs are particularly vulnerable to arterial damage because the arteries are comparatively near the surface. If it does occur and the blood is spurting, a tourniquet should be applied immediately. This can be done by placing a pad on the course of the artery *above* where it has been cut and covering it over with a really tight bandage (*photo 3*). The tightness required can be judged by the pressure needed to stop the bleeding, but never leave the tourniquet on for more than half an hour. Why? Because, with the tourniquet pressing on the artery, the blood supply is stopped to all parts of the limb below the tourniquet. Continued pressure would lead to death of the blood-starved tissues and gangrene would ensue.

Having applied the first-aid, send for your veterinary surgeon immediately. The first half-hour period of the tourniquet application will probably give him time to get there. If not, release the tourniquet for **one minute**, then

28

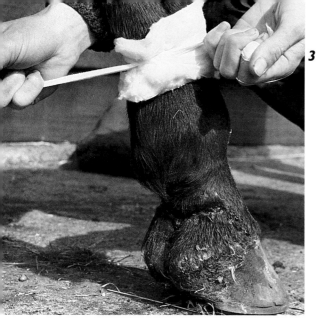

3

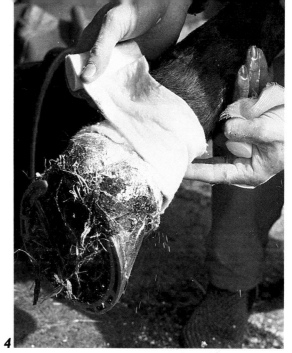

4

re-apply slightly higher up or lower down.

The veterinary surgeon will probably pick up the damaged artery with artery forceps and ligature it. If this has to be done, the smaller arteries in the area enlarge to make up or compensate for the artery that has been lost. This phenomenon is called the development of collateral circulation.

If the haemorrhage is venous, only minimal pressure is required to control it and this pressure can be applied directly by covering the wound with a thick wad of cotton wool and then bandaging over it (*photo 4*).

Veterinary attention, of course, is vital at all times. Not only have the wounds to be

dressed with sulpha drugs or antibiotics and possibly stitched, but an anti-tetanus injection or booster injection is always a wise insurance against the loss of the animal.

In both arteries and veins, nature plays a large part by clotting the blood. In veins these clots quickly seal off the damage, but in arteries the powerful pressure of the pumped arterial blood keeps blowing out the clots.

The golden rule, therefore, is: with all bleeding — from any part of the body — apply first-aid control, then send for your veterinary surgeon immediately.

14
Faults in Conformation

A good blacksmith is worth his weight in gold in the attempted correction of the following conformation faults.

Brushing

Brushing is hitting the inside of a fetlock with

the opposite hoof or shoe. It happens in horses with narrow chests and in those that do not move squarely but 'swing a leg'.

What to do about it

Brushing boots which provide a pad over the

fetlock can be used (*photo 1*). Whilst the brushing boot will prevent damage to the leg, it does nothing to solve or prevent the problem.

Sensible shoeing is a much better idea. **The shoe of the leg that has been struck** should have the inside branch raised. This helps to throw that fetlock a little further out and may just keep it clear when the horse is going on a road or a hard surface. Obviously the raised branch would have little, if any, effect on soft going.

The inside branch of the shoe that is doing the striking should be kept inside the level of the wall (*photo 2*), so that if brushing does occur it will be the wall and not the shoe that does the striking and consequently considerably less damage will be done.

Brushing is due entirely to faulty conformation. Although technically not an unsoundness, it constitutes a serious defect that can prove a nuisance throughout the whole of the horse's life. One should therefore think very carefully before buying a horse that shows evidence of brushing.

Overreach

An overreach almost invariably occurs during jumping or galloping. The hind foot shoe catches the back of the pastern (*photo 3*) or

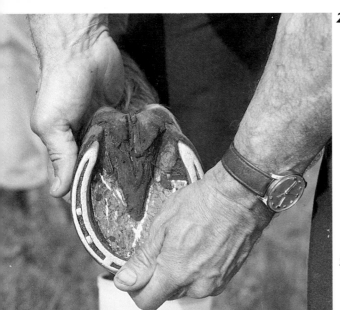

1

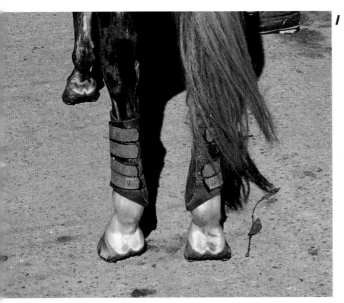

2

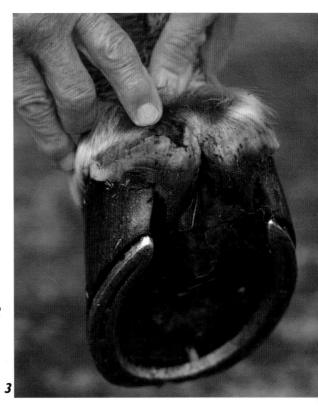

3

the bulb of the heel of the fore foot and cuts it **downward**. This cut may be slight — a graze — or it may be a deep cut involving most of the bulb of the heel.

Heavy going obviously can predispose to overreaching since the horse may have difficulty in pulling his forelegs out of the mud before the hind feet come forward.

Treatment

An overreach wound must have prompt and skilled attention because the downward cut produces a pocket, without drainage, where dirt and infection can quickly gather.

Prevention

Shorten the toes of the hind feet and shoe with light plates. Overreach boots (*photo 4*) should be worn especially when jumping.

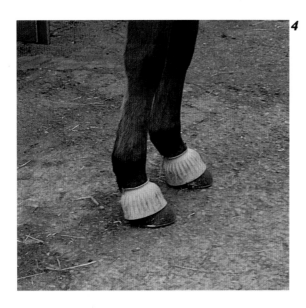

4

Forging

'Forging' or 'clacking' is a less serious form of overreaching where the toe of the hind foot strikes the sole of a fore foot, or the iron of the fore shoe, with a resultant click.

Causes

1. Bad shoeing, e.g., when the toes are left too long.
2. Fatigue or lack of condition.
3. Hereditary fault in the gait (not often seen).

Treatment

A good blacksmith plus some decent feeding.

Speedy cutting

Speedy cutting rarely happens in riding horses. It is most liable to occur in horses with a high action, like the trotting ponies. In many ways it is similar to brushing, but in speedy cutting the part struck is either half way up the inside of the cannon bone or the inside of the knee.

Prevention

Similar to that recommended for brushing, with extra-special attention being paid to the feet and shoes.

15
Stable Vices

Windsucking and crib-biting

A horse can windsuck without crib-biting, but he crib-bites in order to windsuck.

Cause

Stable vices are the result of idleness. They develop in horses kept far too long in the box without exercise, and are due to boredom. They can occur at any age but are usually seen more in older horses simply because they do less work.

Windsucking is drawing the air into the mouth and then forcing it down the gullet into the stomach. When doing this, many horses catch onto the manger, the door or any spar and this is what is known as crib-biting (*photo 1*).

Having got the air into his mouth, he then generally arches his neck quickly as he swallows the air.

Eventually a persistent offender becomes expert and can windsuck without crib-biting.

What effect does it have?

Windsucking upsets the stomach and leads to indigestion, which becomes chronic. Not only does the horse become unthrifty, but he is more liable to develop flatulent colic.

How to spot a windsucker and crib-biter

The teeth are unnaturally worn (*photo 2*). If you suspect unnatural wear, observe the horse patiently and you will see or hear him at it.

Treatment

In many cases treatment is useless but it is always worth trying.

First of all, get the horse into regular work so that when he gets back to his box he is tired and not bored.

Remove everything and anything on which he can bite — manger, spars, etc. — and if you can't remove them soak them in creosote. Keep both halves of the door closed so that there is no exposed edge.

Another treatment, often effective, comprises a strap which is fitted round the neck just behind the ears and passes round the back of the jaw. This strap may be used by itself, as illustrated (*photo 3*), or it may be

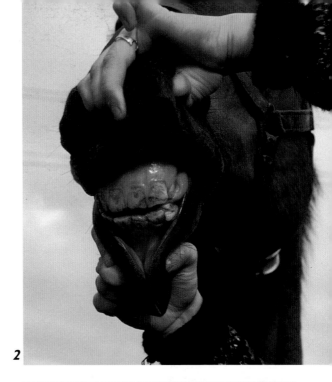

2

3

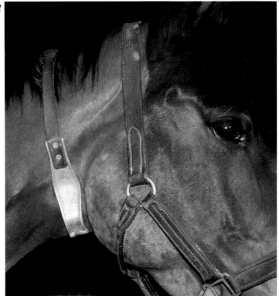

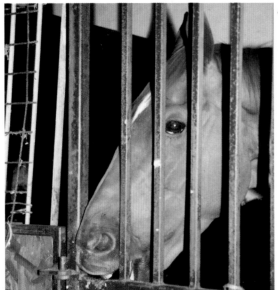

/

threaded through a heart-shaped piece of doubled, very stiff leather. The point of the heart fits in between the angles of the two lower jaws (*photo 4*). When the horse arches his neck to swallow the wind, the point of the heart jags him and forces him to put his head forward and let the wind out of his mouth.

Occasionally with bad cases, a piece of metal, like a steel spring, can be fitted to the

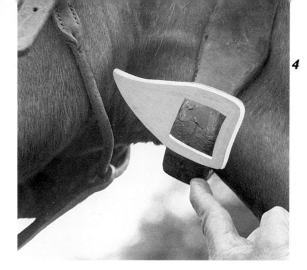

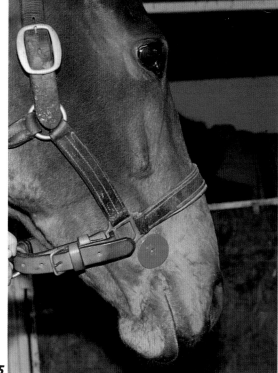

point of the heart.

Some horses quickly learn to manoeuvre the heart out of position. When this happens, put a head collar on and tie the strap in position with pieces of string or a shoelace.

Obviously, any success in treatment by these methods will be slow and the results will largely depend on how long the vice has been present. With persistence and luck, however, even some of the chronic cases can be cured, but there is certainly no guarantee.

There is a simple surgical operation which, in my experience, offers the greatest chance of a rapid and permanent cure.

The operation, first used in Scandinavia, involves making two small permanent holes, one on either side of the horse's mouth. However, the holes, or fistulae as we call them, produce no great disfigurement and are only visible on close examination. The fistulae prevent the formation of the vacuum in the mouth and throat which is necessary for swallowing air.

General anaesthesia is necessary but the technique is amazingly simple. A horizontal 5 cm cut is made over the first cheek teeth. The incision is continued through the muscle and into the mouth. The mucous membrane or lining of the mouth is stiched to the skin to create the permanent fistula. To make sure the fistula does not heal, a small nickel-plated or plastic cannula is stitched into the hole and left for the first six months (*photo 5*). The operation is repeated on the other side.

The one slight snag I have found is that the patients have some difficulty in drinking for the first few days, but they soon adapt themselves. None of them are able to windsuck and they soon give up trying.

I would say that it is most important to catch the windsucking cases as early as possible and to embark on this surgical operation with the utmost confidence.

Prevention

Keep the horse or pony in regular work and soak with creosote all potential biting edges within the box. The creosoting should be repeated every six months.

Just one last word — windsucking and crib-biting are a definite unsoundness and a suspect case should never be purchased without a careful veterinary examination.

Weaving

Weaving is another stable vice and, again, an unsoundness. In other words, never buy a windsucker or a weaver.

Cause

Once again — boredom.

Symptoms

A weaver stands rocking from one fore foot

onto the other, and will often continue to do it for long periods. He will then walk round and start again (*photos 6 & 7*).

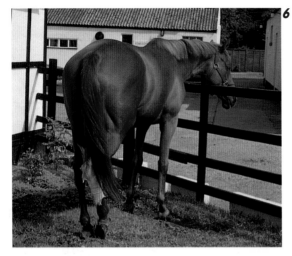

6

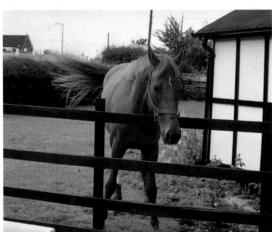

7

Weaving occurs particularly in a box with a half door that opens out into a yard. The horse will stand looking out over the door rocking to and fro. In fact, frequently the floor will be worn in two hollows close to the door. This action makes the horse tired and less capable of hard work.

Treatment
Avoid boredom by keeping the horse or pony in regular hard work, so that when he comes back to the box he is too tired to do anything but sleep. Keep the top half of the box door closed.

If possible, turn him out to grass. Even a bad case will rarely, if ever, weave at grass.

Prevention
If the horse is not in regular hard work, he should be kept at grass or in a paddock.

Polydipsia (Excessive drinking)

Cause
Boredom. A salt lick in the box will often trigger off the habit.

Symptoms
The horse may look well and eat normally but just drinks and urinates continuously for something to do.

Treatment
Restrict the drinking water to a maximum of ten gallons a day and the vice will soon disappear.

16
Saddle and Girth Sores

Saddle sores
Saddle sores are sores that appear on the back under the saddle (*photo 1*). They are due to various faults.

A good-fitting saddle (*photo 2*) must be the correct length for the size of the pony — a reputable saddler is the best person to advise on this.

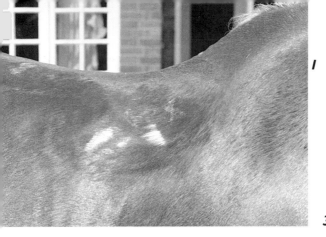

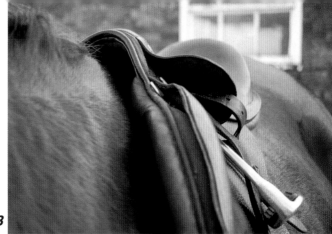

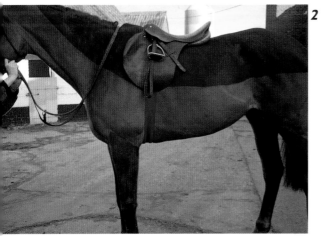

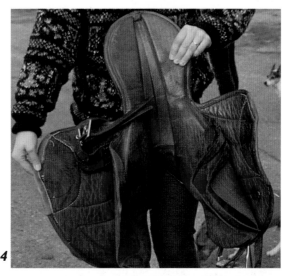

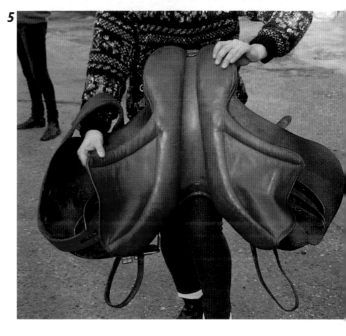

The seat of the saddle should fit smoothly and evenly on the back.

The pommel, i.e. the arch at the front, must be high and well clear of the withers (*photo 3*).

The cannel or tunnel running from the front to the back must be clear, permitting the passage of air and never at any time exerting pressure on the spine.

Sores occur most commonly when the saddle stuffing becomes lumpy or when the saddle lining gets wrinkled or torn (*photo 4*). The lining may be flannel, though good saddles are usually lined with leather or linen (*photo 5*).

The lumpy stuffing or the wrinkled lining produces excessive pressure on a certain point. This inhibits the flow of blood to that part of the skin. Depending on the length of time the pressure is maintained, varying amounts of damage result.

If the condition is spotted early, there will

only be a slight erosion of the skin surface (*photo 6*), but if the pressure is allowed to continue on that point, the skin will die. The affected part will subsequently slough out (or come away) leaving a nasty sore.

Another common cause of saddle sores is dirt. The linings become covered with hair, dried sweat and even mud; and once again, areas of uneven pressure are set up.

Saddle sores, can, of course, be caused simply by bad riding. If you sit in the saddle with more weight on one buttock than the other, or if you persistently roll around in the saddle, then chafing and soreness can soon result. The golden rule, when mounted, is to sit square and sit still.

Girth sores

Once again there are various causes:
1. Old girths that are rough on the inside (*photo 7*).
2. Dirty girths — chafing and producing sores (*photo 8*). Undoubtedly, string girths appear to cause more trouble than those made of leather or webbing.
3. A badly fitting saddle or a saddle set too far forward. The girth will then rub on the skin at the back of the elbows and produce nasty sores. This happens very often with fat ponies freshly off the grass, when it is well-nigh impossible to keep the girths in their correct position.

It is illegal in the UK to ride a horse with a saddle sore or a girth sore, so obviously everything should be done to prevent them.

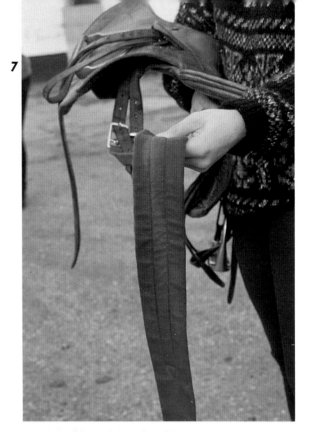

7

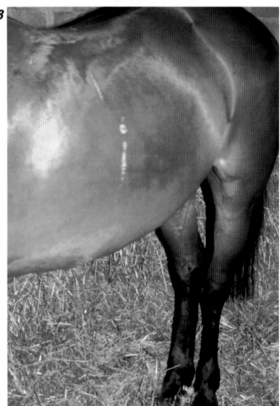

8

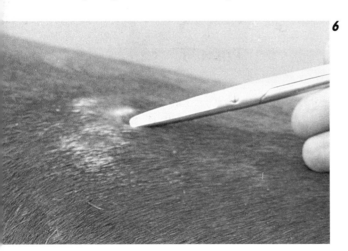

6

How to prevent saddle and girth sores

After the saddle has been put on and girthed up and you are sure it is in the correct position, draw each of the horse's forelegs well forward — get in front and pull them well out (*photo 9*). This brings the skin clear into its correct position below the girth.

Even if the saddle is a perfect fit, and even if it is correctly put on, there is always some slight inhibition of the blood flow through the skin of the back. Obviously, therefore, if you are at a show, gymkhana or on a long hack, you must stop periodically — preferably every hour. Slacken the girth, raise the saddle and allow the blood to flow freely for at least five minutes throughout the pressure area. So often one sees children at shows leaving their ponies tightly girthed up while they go off for ice-cream, tea or to watch the other events. This is very bad. If you have the opportunity of a breather, give your pony's back and sides a breather also.

Make sure that at all times, especially when you move onto a bigger pony or horse, that you have a good fitting saddle and girth. Any experienced horseman should soon put you right, though it is always best to get the opinion of the saddler.

Keep the saddle and girth particularly clean. This means that after every ride both the saddle and girth must be sponged down and dried thoroughly, paying particular attention to the inside linings.

Sit correctly in the saddle (*photo 10*) and don't roll about.

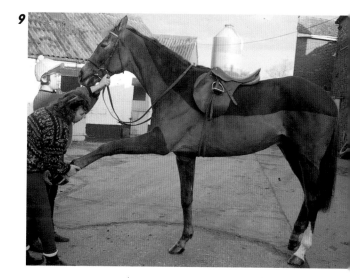

9

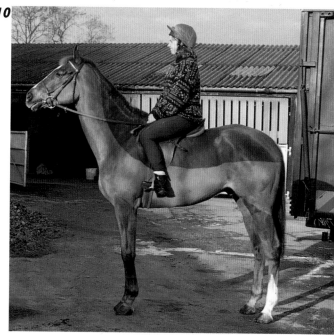

10

Treatment

Treatment depends on the extent of damage but the one thing that is always essential is rest — complete rest. A saddle sore or a girth sore will never heal if it is periodically exposed to further chafing. This is just commonsense and yet the necessity for complete rest is so often disregarded.

There is always some inflammation and the risk of infection, therefore the first dressing may have to be a kaolin poultice containing some antiseptic or preferably some sulphonamide powder. If this type of dressing doesn't remove the pain and inflammation within a day or two, then you should send for your veterinary surgeon. Antibiotics may be needed to combat infection or, if there is a dead portion — what we call 'an area of necrosis' — it may have to be dissected out.

The rest period may extend to several weeks, or even several months, but on no account should the saddle or girth be put on until the wound is completely healed and all trace of tenderness has gone.

When the wound has healed over, but is not

37

yet haired, it is often a good idea to have the saddle 'chambered' by the saddler. He will mark on the saddle lining the position of the unprotected skin. He will then take back the lining and remove some of the stuffing over the marked area. When the lining is replaced, little or no pressure will be exerted on the healed part. This is always well worth doing. A second sore on the same site will take longer to heal than the first.

Photo 11 shows a typical healed lesion.

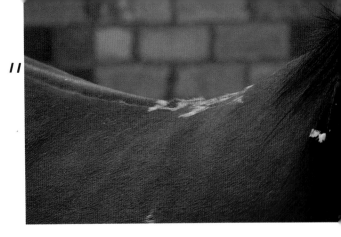

11

17
Feeding

Correct feeding is vitally important. Photo 1 shows an excellent example of a properly fed horse.

In nature, the horse feeds entirely on grass and herbs plus a little earth from which he obtains certain minerals essential to his well-being.

This is sufficient for a horse running wild or during a summer period when he is doing no work. During the winter, however, and also all the year round when in work, a horse requires some additive or extra feed.

The three standard feedingstuffs for horses are hay, oats and bran, and the quantities to be

fed will depend on the amount of work the horse is expected to do.

The most important point to remember is that a horse's stomach (*photo 2*) is very small in proportion to his size. If you watch a horse at grass, you will see he is nibbling away most of the time, resting only for short periods.

2

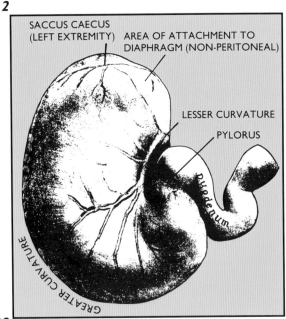

SACCUS CAECUS (LEFT EXTREMITY) AREA OF ATTACHMENT TO DIAPHRAGM (NON-PERITONEAL)

LESSER CURVATURE

PYLORUS

duodenum

GREATER CURVATURE

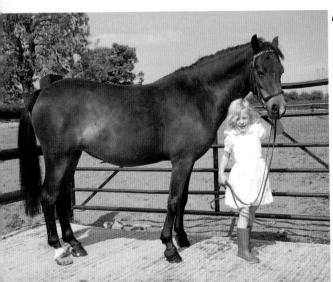

1

The same goes on through the night. Obviously this must be the rigid criterion or guide to the correct feeding of your horse or pony.

Hay

Hay can be available to the horse more or less at all times but it **must be good quality.** Moambray or otherwise damaged hay can cause a great deal of trouble, so always examine the hay before feeding (*photo 3*). Unless very hungry, a horse will not eat bad hay. There is no better judge of the quality of hay than a horse.

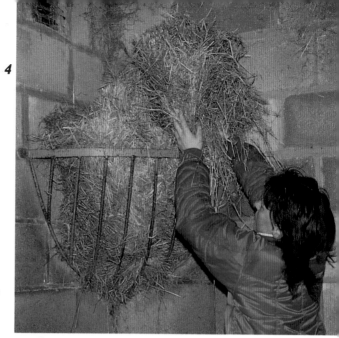

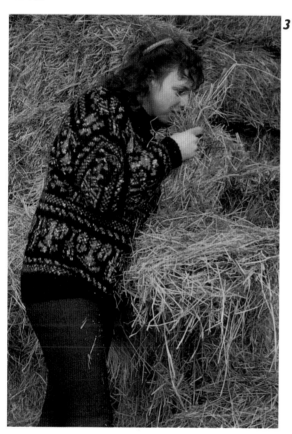

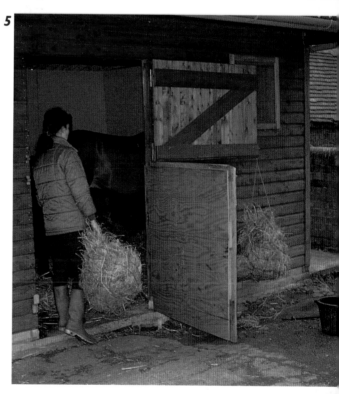

Hay can be fed in three ways:
(a) by just throwing it in the corner of the loose box
(b) in hay racks (*photo 4*)
(c) in hay nets (*photo 5*)
If hay nets are used, they must be placed very high because, as they empty, they become longer and longer and the horse, in pawing at them, may get a leg caught up in the net with disastrous consequences. The horse may get cast and break a leg, or the net may cause a rope burn round the pastern which can leave permanent damage.

Oats

When fed to horses oats should be 'kibbled' or

39

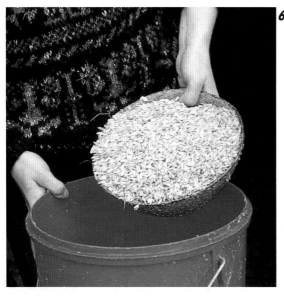

6 bruised (*photo 6*). Whole oats can be fed but many of them pass through the bowel without being digested: this is a foolish waste.

Bran

Bran should never be fed dry if fed alone. The horse may make the dry bran into a ball and this can block his oesophagus causing 'choke'. The bran can be fed either damped (*photo 7*) or mixed with cut or chopped hay. Even when fed with oats, bran should be damped.

Manufacturers are now supplying pony and horse nuts or cubes (*photo 8*). These are generally a compound of hay, oats and bran with perhaps some added maize or barley. It is a very easy way to feed and, in many ways, completely satisfactory. However, it is much more expensive.

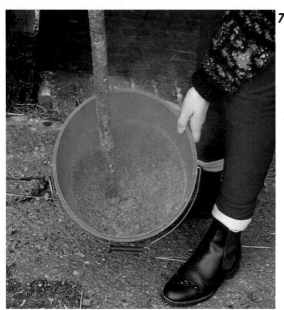

7

Times of feeding

Feeding should be three times a day, stretching the day out as long as possible from early morning to late at night. During the night, leave plenty of hay with the horse so that his stomach never becomes completely empty. In this way you simulate nature and allow the horse to live a more normal life.

Amounts of concentrates to be fed

It is impossible to lay down hard-and-fast rules for the amounts of concentrates to be fed. They depend on the size of the horse and on the amount of work he is going to do.

Water

Without doubt, the most important feed of all is water. Fresh clean water should be with the horse **constantly day and night** so that he can drink as and when he likes.

The water must be clean and fresh **8** (*photo 9*) — not a bucket of liquid manure as one frequently sees.

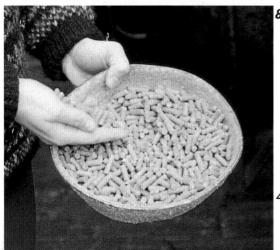

Winter keep

Many pony owners, both adult and young, are full of enthusiasm during the summer while the shows and gymkhanas are on. When the winter comes, however, the pony is frequently turned out into a field without shelter and forgotten. This is not only a sad state of affairs but an absolute disgrace, and such owners

40

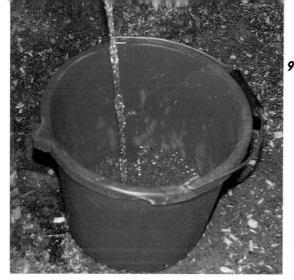

9

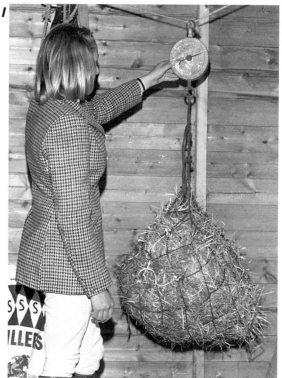

10

11

should be prosecuted for cruelty.

The pony can do well outdoors during the winter provided it has some form of shelter and is well and regularly fed. Without shelter or food the winter is a nightmare for even the toughest of ponies. From the end of September until the beginning of April there is little or no feeding value in the grass, and even this rough herbage gets sparser and sparser every day.

For shelter a decent loose box with an open door is the ideal (*photo 10*), though satisfactory cover can be provided by improvisation of any old farm building.

For winter feeding, the amount needed will depend on whether or not the animal is going to be worked. Some ponies are ridden two or three times a week and even do an odd day's hunting; others are left out all winter and not used until the following spring.

An average 13.2 pony will require a minimum of 10 lb of hay per day. Very few people realise what 10 lb of hay looks like, so the best idea is to weigh a hay net full and work from that (*photo 11*). In addition to the hay, the pony will require feeding night and morning. If it is being worked, it will need roughly 3 lb of bruised or rolled oats and 1 lb of bran per day, split into two feeds. If not working then 3 to 4 lb of damped bran is adequate, again in two feeds.

For variety you can add some boiled turnip, sliced carrot, or a small quantity of boiled linseed (a handful is enough) (*photo 12*) to the feeds. If the weather is very cold, add a good handful of boiled barley.

12

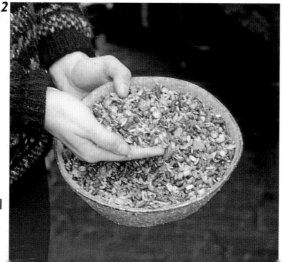

To last the winter, you will require approximately 30 cwt of best quality hay. Remember, only the best hay is good enough for horses. For ponies, ryegrass hay is probably best.

The cost of a winter's keep, including extras like carrots, barley, etc., will probably be considerable. Any hobby, however, costs money, and unless you are prepared to spend on first-class food, plus shoeing and veterinary bills, then it is much better not to start keeping a pony.

Two other important points. During the winter, even though the pony is turned out, his feet require regular attention. Every four to six weeks the blacksmith will have to be called in.

Finally, water — you must keep checking the drinking water. If there is a frost, the water supply may freeze over and the ice will have to be broken three or four times a day. If necessary, give your pony buckets of clean fresh water, and at all times make sure he has plenty.

PROBLEMS ASSOCIATED WITH FEEDING

Thick cloudy urine

Perhaps the most common dietetic upset seen in horses is the passing of thick cloudy urine (*photo 13*). The patient may also have some difficulty in urinating.

Cause
Cloudy urine is due to eating mouldy hay or to eating damp bedding. The latter bad habit can be triggered off by a mineral deficiency, probably a shortage of phosphorus.

Treatment and prevention
Provide best quality hay. If the bedding is being eaten, bed down with sawdust or peat moss and provide a mineral lick containing phosphorus as a trace element, plus a daily bran mash.

Coprophagy

Just occasionally a horse will persistently eat his own dung. This condition is called coprophagy

and is seen mostly in stabled horses (*photo 14*).

Cause
A deficiency of vitamin B, especially vitamin B_1.

Symptoms
Apart from the obvious, the patient will most likely be unthrifty not only because of the vitamin deficiency but also because he will continually re-infect himself with roundworms, producing a fair degree of anaemia.

Treatment
Intravenous or intramuscular injections of vitamin B compound combined with oral iron and vitamin supplements. Also regular worming every six weeks.

Most important of all during treatment is to prevent the patient from reaching the dung by tying him up.

13

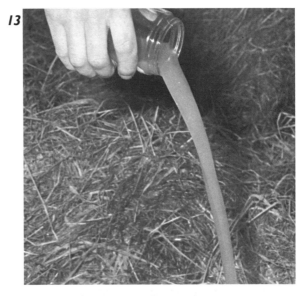

14

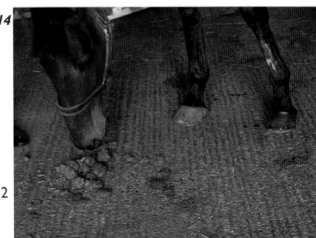

42

General Diseases and Conditions

18
Parasites

A parasite is an organism or creature that lives on or in an animal entirely at that animal's expense. The animal on or in which the parasite lives is called the host.

There are two main types of parasites:

(a) External, which live on the surface of the animal.

(b) Internal, which live inside the animal.

EXTERNAL PARASITES

Sarcoptic mange

This is the most serious of the diseases caused by external equine parasites, but fortunately it has been largely eliminated in the United Kingdom. Sarcoptic mange is a notifiable disease, i.e. the Police and Ministry of Agriculture have to be informed if there is any suspicious or confirmed case.

Method of spread

Sarcoptic mange is a contagious disease. However, although a horse may be near an affected one, it will not contract it unless the two rub against one another. This is because horse mange, as in other animals, is caused by mites (*see illustration*). Of course, the mites

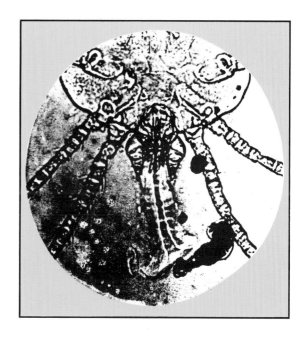

can also be picked up from loose boxes, grooming tackle, fence posts, etc.

Symptoms

Intense irritation and itching. It can start anywhere but often flares up first at the tail, head, legs or at the base of the mane. The horse or pony bites or rubs the part almost continuously; very soon bald patches will appear.

Diagnosis and treatment
Your veterinary surgeon should be consulted in all suspect cases. He will take skin scrapings and examine them under the microscope. If positive, he will report the case to the authorities, who will quarantine the animal and supervise the thorough disinfection of the box, bridles, saddlery and grooming equipment.

He will supply baths or dressings which will need to be applied every week for at least a month to cope with the mite eggs as they continue to hatch out. If the horse is long-coated, it will have to be clipped.

If the skin scrapings are negative, the veterinary surgeon will prescribe the correct treatment for the condition.

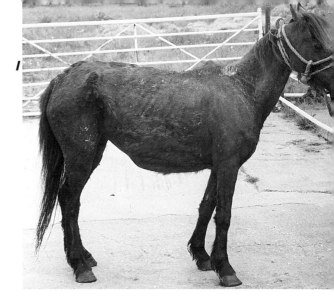

Lice

These are undoubtedly the most common of the external horse parasites (*photo 1*). Often, after castrating a colt, my arms and gown have been covered with them.

Method of spread
Lice are picked up in the same way as the mange mites, viz. by direct contact or via dirty boxes, tackle, etc. Like mange, it is a contagious condition.

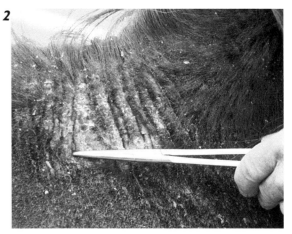

Symptoms
Identical to mange in the early stages, i.e. rubbing, biting and bare patches. However, close examination by a veterinary surgeon or by a reasonably knowledgeable horseman will show the lice and the minute white louse eggs (*photo 2*) situated at varying distances along the hair shafts.

Lice are seen chiefly on horses that are badly fed and neglected, and are more common on the long-coated than the clipped out, simply because the clipped-out animal is usually regularly fed and carefully groomed.

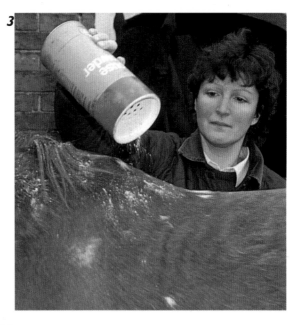

Treatment
There are many good lice baths and louse powders (*photo 3*), any one of which will kill

the adult lice. However, as in mange, the dressings do not kill the eggs and therefore must be repeated once a week for several weeks to catch the lice as they hatch out and before they have a chance to lay more eggs.

Prevention
Remember: A well-cared for horse will never get lice. Good, regular feeding, regular exercise and grooming will nearly always prevent the establishment of a lice infestation.

INTERNAL PARASITES

In horses, as in most other animals, there are two main types of worms:
1. Flat worms, known as tapeworms.
2. Roundworms.

Tapeworms

The tapeworm is described as a 'commensal' because it does not do any damage to the horse's intestines. It merely eats the food that has been digested and passed into the intestine for absorption. The simple result is that the horse does not get the full benefit from the food he is eating and he loses condition (*photo 4*).

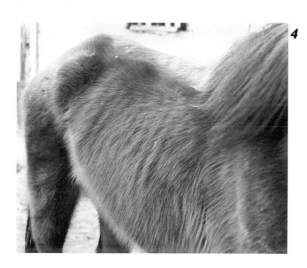

4

Life history
The tapeworm lays eggs in its tail, then detaches the egg-laden tail, which is passed out onto the pastures.
The eggs hatch out into minute larvae which

are eaten by small non-parasitic mites. Inside the mites the larvae develop into cysts.
The horse eats the mites with the grass and, in the horse's intestine, the cysts rupture and develop very quickly into adult tapeworms — male and female — which copulate and start the cycle once more *(see diagram A)*.

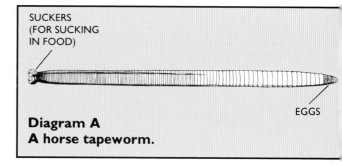

SUCKERS (FOR SUCKING IN FOOD)

EGGS

Diagram A
A horse tapeworm.

Roundworms

There are several different types of roundworms. They affect horses much more frequently than tapeworms do and cause a great deal more serious damage.
The common roundworms may vary in size from minute threads to up to three inches long *(see diagram B)*, whereas the less common horse ascarids can be up to one foot in length.

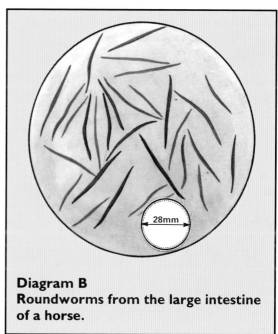

28mm

Diagram B
Roundworms from the large intestine of a horse.

Can all horses be affected?

All horses can be affected with roundworms, but undoubtedly young horses are more susceptible and in them the damage is greatest. The older horses acquire varying degrees of immunity.

Roundworms are passed by 'carrier' horses which may show no apparent signs of infestation. The young susceptible horses pick up the infection from the pastures.

The worms are cast out in the dung of the 'carrier' or infected animal. They pass through three developmental larva forms but only the third form is infective.

The infective larvae are eaten by another horse. They travel to the intestines (or bowels) and there they migrate through the bowel wall to many parts of the body. Needless to say, during their journeyings the larvae can cause great damage. For example in arteries they can completely block the flow of blood producing ballooning of the arterial walls which causes aneurisms. They can rupture the walls of the blood vessels and cause haemorrhages which may prove fatal; and damage the liver, the lungs and any other organ in the body (see diagram C). Migration of the larvae in the legs can produce swellings, especially in foals.

When they finally return to the intestines they attach themselves to the bowel lining by teeth and suck blood (*photo 5*). (Hence the 'red' worms you often see in the dung.) They therefore produce anaemia. Photo 6 shows the white gums of a horse heavily infected with roundworms. Contrast these with the pink gums of a healthy horse in photo 7.

5

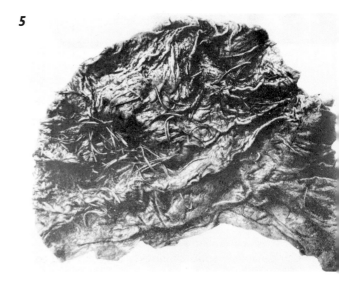

6

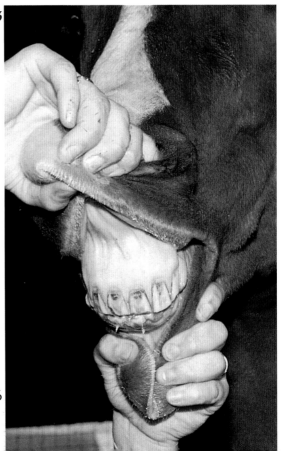

Diagram C
Roundworms on the surface of the mucosa of the large intestine of a horse.

46

Roundworms can also cause irritation of the bowel leading to colicky pains, acute enteritis, diarrhoea (*photo 8*) and even death.

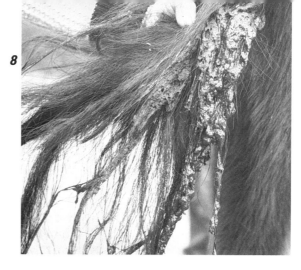

8

How to spot worms

An unthrifty young horse, particularly when at grass, should always be suspect. Your veterinary surgeon can and will estimate the degree of infestation by examining the droppings microscopically (*photo 9*).

It is a good idea to get your veterinary surgeon to carry this out regularly twice a year, particularly with the young horses.

Prevention

Dose the horses every six weeks — with a reputable anthelmintic (*photo 10*). Start dosing a foal at two months of age. But one simple preventive precaution which is well worth trying is to lift the droppings every day. This may not be practical, but it is obviously an effective way of controlling infection, especially if, as in many cases, the horses dung in a particular corner.

Avoid continued intensive grazing of comparatively small paddocks. This can lead to

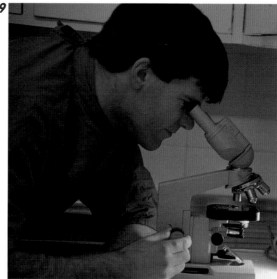

9

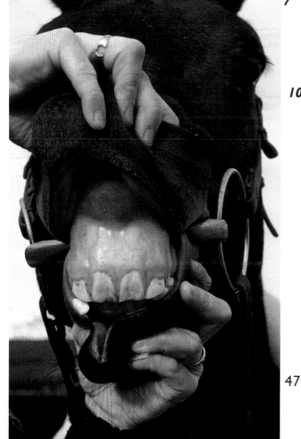

7

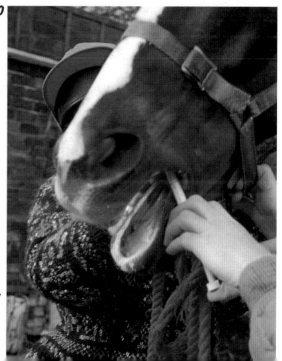

10

a massive build-up of roundworms — a build-up so gross that it may defy all attempts at control by treatment and may lead to widespread deaths.

Use small paddocks only occasionally, e.g. for foaling.

Treatment

In badly affected cases, treatment is very much a job for your veterinary surgeon.

After estimating and identifying the worms, he will stomach pump a maximum dose of the appropriate anthelmintic into the patient (*photo 11*), and will usually prescribe iron and vitamin B_{12} injections for the anaemia and debility.

Recent scientific work has shown that six-weekly dosing is necessary to keep horses *completely* free from worm effects. Though this may not always be practical, it is as well to bear the fact in mind, particularly during the grazing season. Such repeated dosing may allow certain roundworms to develop a tolerance to a particular anthelmintic, so it is a good idea to ring the changes with the drug used. There are a number of excellent products available.

Lungworms and filarial worms

Lungworms live most of their lives in the bronchial tubes and can cause coughing though they are much more of a menace in donkeys. Most modern anthelmintics act against the horse lungworm larvae.

Minute thread worms called filarial worms may be found inside the eyes or in the skin; such infections are for the veterinary surgeon to diagnose and treat.

TWO OTHER PARASITES

There are two other parasites, both part of the life cycle of flies.

Bott fly

The bott fly appears in fields roughly from June till September. It is very similar in appearance in many ways to the ordinary bumble bee but it cannot bite or sting. It does, however, lay its eggs on the tips of the hairs of the forelegs, generally on the cannon bone or just above the knee on the inside (*photo 12*).

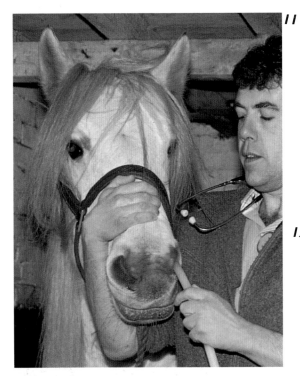

11

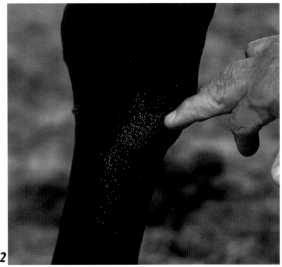

12

This fly is particularly noticeable in warm summer weather, and horses often become agitated when it is around.

The eggs hatch into small larvae which the horse licks into his mouth. There the larvae burrow into the tongue or cheeks and remain there for two or three weeks without apparently causing any worry.

From the mouth they migrate to the stomach by coming out from their burrows and being swallowed. In the stomach they develop into larger larvae and, by means of their teeth, attach themselves to the inside of the stomach wall (*photo 13*). They eat the horse's food and produce a slight gastritis in the area where they are holding on. If the botts are in large numbers, this area may be extensive and occasionally the botts partially occlude the passage of food.

They stay in the stomach all winter, and in the following spring (usually about May) they release their hold, pass out with the dung and develop into adult flies.

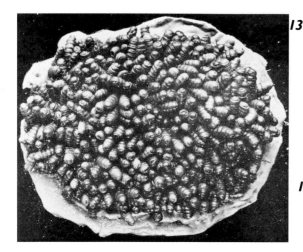
13

Symptoms
In small numbers they appear to cause little trouble, but in heavy infestations the horse may be unthrifty, show a capricious appetite and may even exhibit recurrent colic.

Treatment
This is very much a job for a veterinary surgeon. Carbon bisulphide, Trichlorfon and Dichlorvos are the drugs of choice. The first two are best administered by stomach pump, and the Equigard should be used exactly as instructed by the manufacturers. Modern dispensers containing anti-bott drugs can be supplied by your veterinary surgeon.

Prevention
Throughout the fly period, brush the eggs off

the forelegs every day. If this is done, the odd few larvae that reach the horse's stomach will do little or no harm.

Warble fly

The warble fly is not nearly so common in the horse as in cattle, but when it does get onto the horse it can cause considerable pain and damage.

Like the bott, the warble fly likes warm weather and appears in the summertime. The eggs are laid at the *base* of the hairs and on the lower parts of all *four* legs. There the eggs hatch out into minute larvae which penetrate the skin and migrate throughout the body till they eventually arrive at the back, frequently just under the saddle area.

They appear as small painful lumps under the skin of the back (*photo 14*). In cattle the mature larvae pass out through the skin to develop into a new generation of flies, but in horses the larvae often die under the skin producing either an abscess or a fistula. When this happens they have to be removed by surgical means (*photo 15*).

Even after surgery, a painful sore remains

14
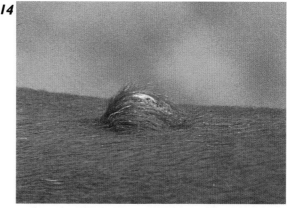

15
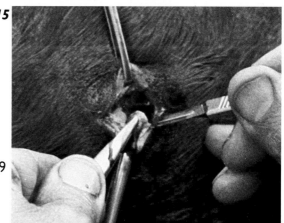

which may take a considerable time to heal sufficiently for the horse to be put back to work.

Prevention and treatment
Prevention in the horse is possible if the horse is at livery on a farm where the cattle are strictly dressed against the fly. Fortunately cattle dressing is now compulsory in Britain.

As for treatment, it must be left to your veterinary surgeon to decide whether surgical removal is necessary. In the majority of cases they are best left severely alone, provided the horse can be adequately rested.

19
Ringworm

Ringworm (*photo 1*) in the horse is a contagious disease.

Cause
A fungus.

How a horse becomes affected
The disease is the result of direct contact with an infected or a 'carrier' horse. A 'carrier' is an animal which transmits the fungus without showing any clinical signs of the disease. Recovered animals sometimes remain 'carriers'. The horse may also pick up the fungus from an infected loose-box or trailer (*photo 2*) or from infected grooming kit, horse blankets, saddles, etc.

1

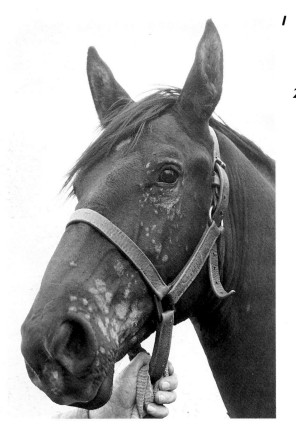

2

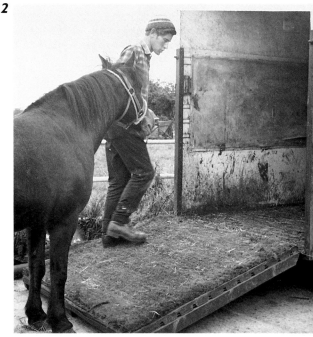

Symptoms

First of all, the hair will appear to stand up and rise in small, irritant circular patches (*photo 3*). The horse may rub the affected area against fence posts, etc.

Then the hair in the patches will fall out and leave circular bald areas. These spots may eventually become crusty or septic.

The fungi that cause ringworm are aerobes, i.e. they require oxygen, so that when the lesions become crusted over, the ones in the centre die and the live fungi keep working outwards away from the centre, thereby producing the typical ringworm. The fungi are therefore to be found in greatest concentration at the outside or periphery of the circular areas.

Diagnosis is made on the symptoms but it can be confirmed definitely only by the examination of skin scrapings in a laboratory.

to remove the crusts and expose the fungi to the effects of the dressing.

One important point to remember: horse ringworm is infectious to man, so be very careful with your hands and nails. Always wear rubber gloves when grooming the infected animal (*photo 5*) and keep the gloves soaking in the disinfectant with the grooming tackle.

A food supplement containing an anti-fungal drug is marketed under the proprietary name of Fulcin. This acts through the bloodstream and I have found it to be a most valuable and effective treatment. The majority of horse owners prefer this internal treatment.

4

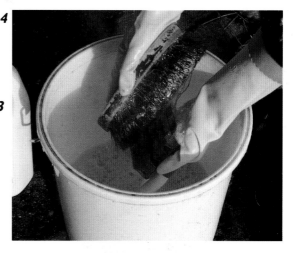

3

5

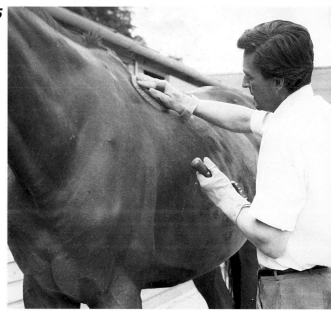

Treatment

An affected or suspect pony or horse should be isolated.

All grooming equipment, rugs, feeding utensils, etc., must be regularly disinfected (*photo 4*) and kept for that specific animal only.

The lesions should be dressed once a week for three weeks, using a reliable non-irritant anti-fungal application which will be supplied by your veterinary surgeon. It is a good idea first to scrub the lesions with hot water and soda

20
Other Irritant Skin Conditions

Tail rubbing or itchy tail

This is a comparatively common condition in ponies and horses of all ages in Britain, particularly during the summer.

Symptoms

These are unmistakable — the horse starts rubbing the base of his tail against gateways or fence posts. The affected areas become bald (*photo 1*), and if rubbing is continued, the skin may become red raw.

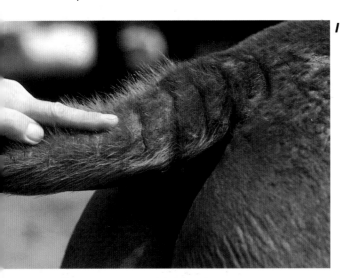

1

Cause

It is usually due to a normally innocuous mange mite, called the chorioptes or symbiotes, which apparently becomes active in the tail only in warm weather, especially if the horse sweats around the root of the tail. However, certain species of roundworms cause severe itching as they wriggle out through the anus and they too produce identical symptoms.

Occasionally, itchy tail can be caused by an allergic condition associated with the eating of certain grass proteins or weeds. It can, of course, be due to sweet itch.

Treatment

Get your veterinary surgeon on the job at once. He will check the faeces for roundworm eggs and will examine the area for mange mites.

When due to mites, I have found that the most satisfactory treatment is the daily application of a 10 per cent solution of benzyl benzoate in surgical spirit (your veterinary surgeon will supply this). The application should not be rubbed in — merely applied soaked into cotton wool, once a day for fourteen days (*photo 2*).

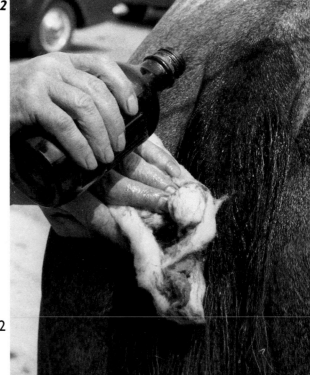

2

Arsenical skin tonic injections, arsenical oral preparations given in the food, and cortisone injections and tablets, all help greatly to improve the condition, but prolonged treatment with these can become very expensive.

In hot weather, box the horse or pony in a cool atmosphere during the day. This avoids the tail sweating and reduces the chance of a digestive allergy.

Have the faeces checked regularly for roundworm eggs and dose accordingly.

Sweet itch

Sweet itch is an irritating disease affecting the withers and quarters of horses and ponies.

Cause
A midge called the *Culicoides pulicaris* that bites the horse or pony on the withers and haunches from April to October, **but only for an hour or so before and after sunset.**

Symptoms
Certain horses seem more susceptible than others, and sweet itch appears to affect only 2-3 per cent of the equine population. Persistent itching occurs along the root of the mane from the withers to the poll (*photo 3*) and also on the back towards the tail. The patient will often rub the parts raw throughout the summer months.

Treatment
All the treatments described for tail rubbing can be tried, but it is much simpler and better to prevent the condition. If the sweet itch does develop, corticosteroid injections and local applications are probably the most effective treatment.

Prevention
Stable the horse or pony that is known to be susceptible at **4 pm every day** from 1st April to the 31st October, and turn him out again either late at night or early next morning.

In the stable or loose box hang several insecticide strips and renew and replace these several times throughout the season. Even better, though rather more expensive, are Aerovap insect killers or other similar installations (*photo 4*).

4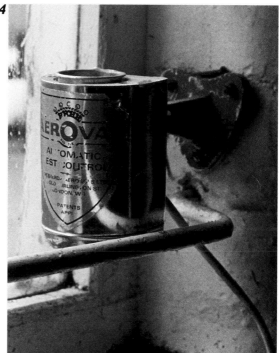

3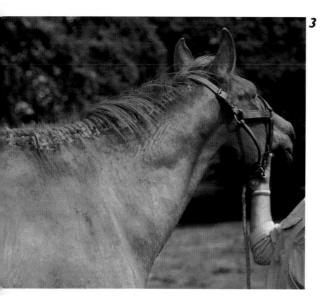

Recent research has shown that local weekly or twice weekly dressings throughout the danger period with a drug called permethrin is a valuable aid in control. The veterinary surgeon will supply you with the necessary 4 per cent solution together with instructions for use.

Itchy legs (Chorioptic mange)

Cause
Mange mites called the chorioptes or symbiotes, similar to those causing itchy tail. On the legs the chorioptes may lie dormant in the apparently normal skin and flare up only when the horse's resistance is lowered.

Symptoms
The patient starts biting his leg or legs and scaly or moist sores rapidly develop (*photo 5*).

Treatment
A gammexane bath scrubbed into the legs with a hard bristle brush. Repeat twice at seven-day intervals.

Prevention
Keep your horse in good condition all the year round.

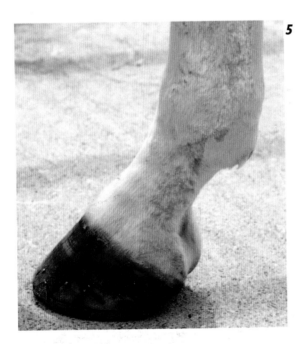

5

Urticaria or 'blane'

This is an allergic condition and is occasionally known as 'nettle-rash'. It is very difficult to describe exactly what is meant by the term 'allergy' but, generally speaking, an allergy occurs when some external factor disagrees with some normal factor within the animal. For example, stings from certain plants (nettles, etc — *photo 6*), or from flies and insects, or through changes in feeding, particularly when protein increase causes indigestion.

Urticaria is not generally serious but it can be very alarming. Usually in veterinary practice it comes through as a panic call and almost invariably by the time we get there the symptoms have subsided.

Symptoms
Raised blotches or weals over the entire body, usually most marked around the head and neck (*photo 7*) and under the belly and tail. Occasionally the head and throat regions swell to twice the normal size and the horse may have difficulty in breathing freely. The temperature and pulse usually remain normal.

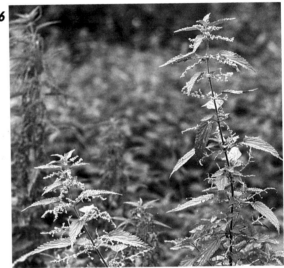

6

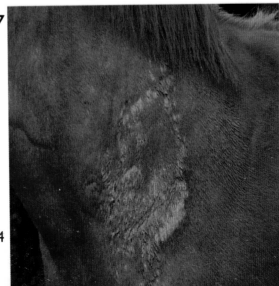

7

54

Treatment
Left alone, the weals will almost invariably die down in a short time. However, there are antihistamine and cortisone injections which appear to clear the condition miraculously.

Acne

Symptoms
Small hard lumps or pimples seen mostly on the skin of the neck (*photo 8*), shoulders and quarters.

Cause
Bacterial infection of the hair follicles; infection can be spread by grooming.

Treatment
A course of antibiotic injections combined with sterilisation of grooming tools. The affected areas should be rubbed over with a fresh clean cloth daily until the lumps have disappeared.

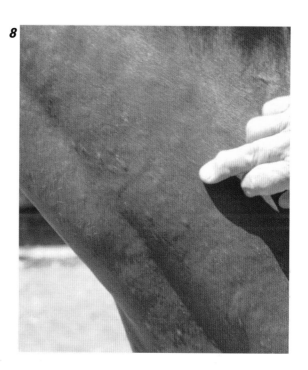

8

21
Tetanus or Lockjaw

This disease is one of the greatest potential enemies of the horse, pony, mule and donkey.

Cause
The germ *Clostridium tetani* — called a sporulating germ because it surrounds itself with a thick protective coat to form what the scientist describes as a 'spore'. The illustration to the right shows sporulating tetanus bacilli in a stained microscopic slide of pus.

The tetanus spore can lie dormant in the ground for many years provided it has available a minimal amount of moisture. For this reason the germ is more often found on moist arable or heavy land than on old, light, dry permanent pasture.

Method of infection
A deep punctured wound provides the ideal

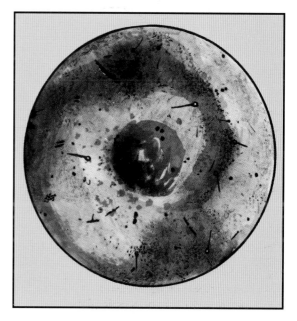

spot for the tetanus spores to get to work (*photo 1*). In such a wound there is little or no

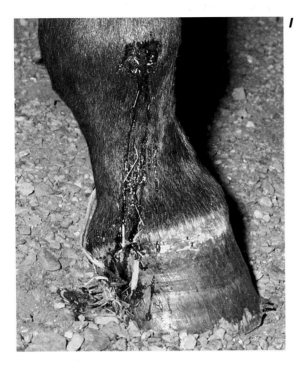

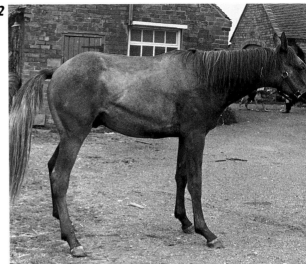

air and the spores, being what we call anaerobes (i.e. germs that dislike oxygen or air), will throw off their protective coats and start to multiply on the spot. The germs do not enter the bloodstream, but they excrete a poisonous waste product called a toxin. This toxin travels from the nerve endings along the nerves towards the spinal column, playing havoc with the nerve's true functions. The resulting symptoms vary according to the amount of toxin and the extent of the nerve involvement.

Symptoms

The first sign usually seen in horses is that the head is poked forward and the nostrils slightly distended giving the muzzle a square appearance (*photo 2*).

The legs are placed slightly wider than normal, particularly the hind legs, with the hocks turned outwards and the tail raised. When made to move the animal walks stiffly as though afraid.

When the back of the hand is brought up sharply against the bottom of the lower jaw

(*photo 3*), the third eyelid (the membrana nictitans) may flash across the eye. This is absolutely diagnostic of tetanus.

As the symptoms advance, the horse may become wildly excited. He may have great difficulty in breathing and the jaws may become firmly clamped with the facial muscles rigid and hard. Needless to say, when this happens the patient is unable to eat or drink.

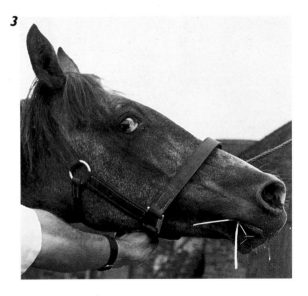

Treatment

Treatment is rarely successful, especially if the symptoms are at all advanced. The patient should be kept as quiet as possible in a dark box. In most cases euthanasia is indicated, but the veterinary surgeon is the person to confirm the diagnosis and make the final decision. Acute cases die or have to be slaughtered immediately. The majority of less severe cases die in five to ten days. If they go over ten days and can still eat, they stand a chance of recovery though it takes a long time.

Prevention

This is one disease which should always be immunised against (*photo 4*). Fortunately highly efficient injections against tetanus are available. The one called Thorovax has the advantage of not producing a local reaction a the injection site.

The best method of control is to have the animals injected with two doses of vaccine at monthly intervals, and a booster dose every

year thereafter. This is the ideal routine and should be followed religiously by every horse or pony owner.

In addition, whenever there is a punctured wound an injection of tetanus antitoxin should also be given by the veterinary surgeon. This gives immediate protection and doubles the insurance.

BOTULISM AND MALIGNANT OEDEMA

Apart from the clostridium bacterium which causes tetanus there are two other dangerous clostridial germs:

Clostridium botulinum

The toxins of this cause the fatal disease botulism.

Source of infection

Forage containing the botulinum toxins from the bodies of dead rodents.

Symptoms

Debility, nerve paralysis, difficulty in chewing and swallowing followed by respiratory paralysis and death.

Clostridium septique

Just occasionally a wound contaminant produces equally virulent toxins which cause malignant oedema leading to extensive oedema (dropsy) of the neck, brisket and abdomen and death in one to four days.

It is my experience that neither of these two conditions is common in the horse.

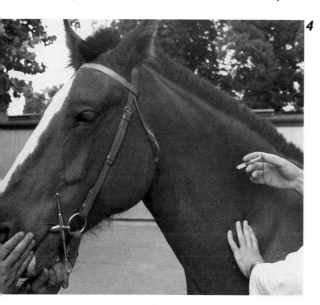

4

22
Transit Tetany

This is a condition which produces symptoms very similar to tetanus. However, transit

tetany can be treated and cured, so it is extremely important to recognise it and to consult a veterinary surgeon immediately.

Animals affected
It can occur in any horse after a prolonged road, rail, sea or plane journey, but is seen mainly in old mares or newly weaned foals that have been rounded up off the mountains, transported by road to markets, and then subsequently to different parts of the country (*photo 1*).

Symptoms
The nostrils wrinkle and the jaw locks. The patient starts to stagger and sweat and is unable to pass urine. When forced to move he exhibits an exaggerated high-pacing gait. The temperature may rise to 105°F (40.5°C) and the pulse is accelerated. The symptoms are alarming and if the condition is not treated promptly and correctly, it can prove fatal.

Treatment
Calcium is the important drug. Your veterinary surgeon will inject it, in solution into the vein

and underneath the skin. He will probably also inject a muscle relaxant and an antibiotic.

Recovery is spectacular. Within one hour the animal will stale normally and start to eat again.

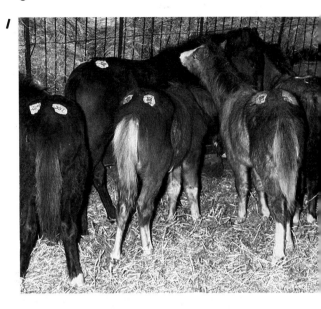

1

23
Purpura Haemorrhagica

The specific cause is unknown though it is probably a plant allergy. Some scientists claim a virus may be involved because the onset of purpura often coincides with lowered resistance. For example, it may flare up when the horse is apparently recovering from strangles or a severe cold. In such cases the allergies may be between the antibodies in the blood and the protein of the bacteria or virus; or there may be a poisonous effect from the bacterial toxins.

Symptoms
The first sign noticed is generally the appearance of a swelling or swellings on the

brisket, along the floor of the belly or on any, or all, of the four legs, usually at the top (*photo 1*).

The purpura swellings or lumps are characteristic in that they have square edges. They are non-painful and pit on pressure.

The temperatures rises several degrees but may drop back to normal or sub-normal after a few days. The pulse is accelerated.

Occasionally the head is affected and the nose swells up (*photo 2*).

Inside the nostrils petechiae (minute red haemorrhages) appear. Similar petechiae occur throughout the entire body, and there may be a bloody or pink coloured discharge from the

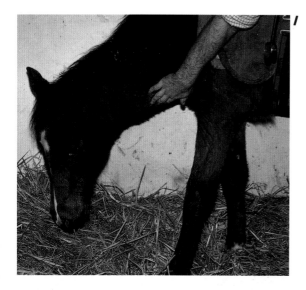

nostrils and from the natural openings (*photo 3*).

The horse is usually extremely sick and may refuse to eat or drink.

Treatment

There is no known specific cure, and the condition is often fatal. However, there are many lines of treatment and some animals do recover, so your veterinary surgeon should be consulted immediately. If the horse keeps eating, its chances of recovery are enhanced though invariably convalescence is prolonged.

It has been my experience, however, that complete recovery from purpura haemorrhagica takes a comparatively long time. My best results have followed blood transfusions combined with antihistamine, steroid and antibiotic injections.

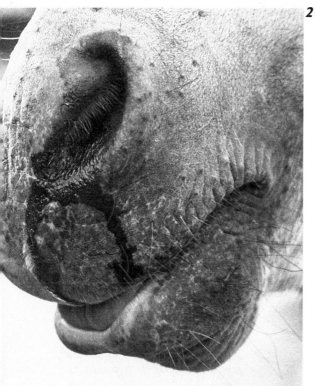

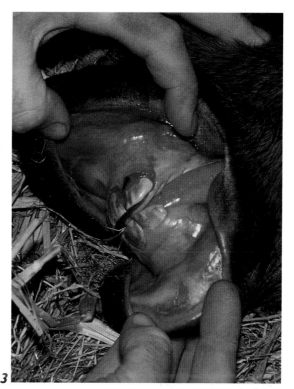

24
Photosensitisation

This is an eczematous skin condition seen occasionally in the unpigmented skin of coloured or grey horses.

Cause
A hypersensitivity to sunlight triggered off usually by the ingestion of excess clover or certain plants and weeds. Occasionally it can flare up as a drug allergy.

Symptoms
Patches of moist eczema breaking out in different parts of the body. If unchecked the affected skin may die and slough off (*photo 1*). If large areas of the body are involved there may be an initial shock effect causing high temperature (105-106°F, 40.5-41°C), rapid pulse and staggering gait.

Treatment
Bring the patient into a cool dark loose box and keep him there till the condition is cured.

Your veterinary surgeon will probably treat with antihistamine and/or cortisone injections and local applications.

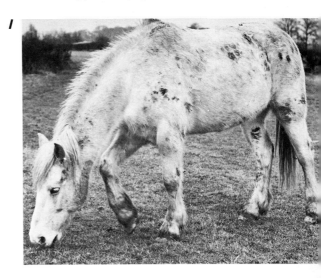

1

25
Melanoma

This condition occurs almost exclusively in grey or white horses. It comprises small growths which spread slowly but insidiously and are nearly always malignant.

Symptoms
Usually multiple small hard lumps develop around the anus and tail base (*photos 1 & 2*). For a considerable while they cause little or no discomfort unless they ulcerate. However, they may continue to spread inside involving the tissues of the pelvic region. The swellings there produce pressure on the obturator and other nerves and lead to an incurable lameness,

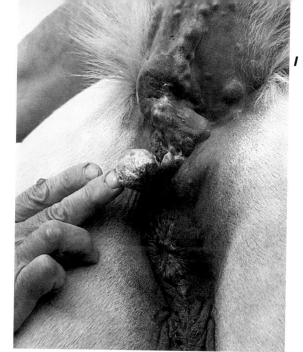

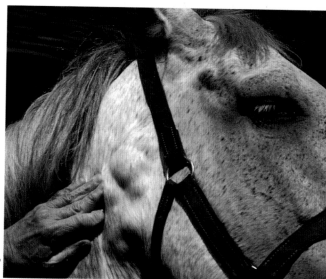

1 which necessitates painless euthanasia.

These tumours also frequently affect the parotid salivary gland (below and in front of the ear) (*photo 3*) and may at times be found in the region of the penis, sheath, udder and occasionally on the legs.

Persistent hind leg lameness in a grey or white horse should always be regarded as possibly due to an internal malignant melanoma.

Treatment
There is none. Your veterinary surgeon will be required to diagnose the internal melanoma, and will advise accordingly. When the growths are external and causing no discomfort or lameness, they should be left severely alone.

2

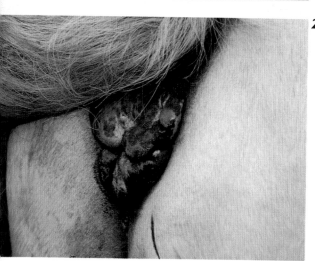

3

26
Cancer

Apart from the melanoma already dealt with and an occasional malignant surface tumour, the only other reasonably common type of cancer I have seen in the horse is the variety known as lymphosarcoma affecting the mesenteric lymph glands which service the intestine.

If allowed to progress such cancer invades the bowel wall producing a marked thickening.

Lymphosarcoma can occur at any age.

Symptoms

A capricious appetite and a progressive loss in condition to the point of acute emaciation (*photo 1*).

Intermittent or persistent diarrhoea develops in the later stages.

Diagnosis

Very much a job for the veterinary surgeon. He will eliminate other possible causes such as teeth, parasites, kidney damage and TB and will send blood samples for profile examination. Unfortunately the blood evidence is not always satisfactory and an exploratory laparotomy may be necessary (i.e. he may have to open into the abdomen).

Treatment

Immediate euthanasia.

CUSHING'S SYNDROME

A much rarer type of cancer — in fact, the case illustrated (*photo 2*) is the only one I have seen in over 50 years of veterinary practice. The cancer or tumour occurs in the pituitary gland at the base of the brain, producing what is known as Cushing's syndrome.

Symptoms

Excess drinking, weight loss and the development of a thick curly coat. Any infection (in this case a foot abscess) fails to respond to treatment.

Treatment

Euthanasia.

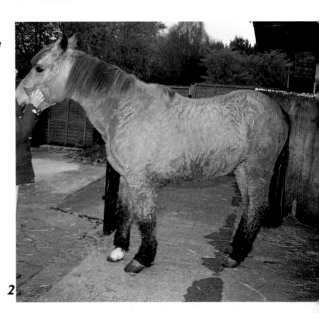

1

2

27
Tuberculosis

Since TB has now been eradicated from British cattle, cases in the horse are rare. Nonetheless I have seen several and the symptoms and treatment are identical to those for lymphosarcoma. The TB lesions first appear in the horse's spleen.

28
Warts and Angleberries

As with all animals, warts on horses and ponies (*photos 1 & 2*) are a nuisance, to say the least, especially during the summer when the flies seek them out for special attention. The persistent irritation of the fly bites makes the animal restless and bad tempered. When the weight of the warts causes them to hang down, they are known as angleberries, especially when they occur around the genital organs.

Causes

It is now fairly well established that warts are caused by viruses. The viruses have not yet been identified, but vaccines can be prepared against them.

Treatment

Even the smallest wart or group of warts should be treated without delay. Modern wart dressings (*photo 3*) are extremely effective provided the mass is not overwhelming. The appropriate dressing will be supplied by your veterinary surgeon.

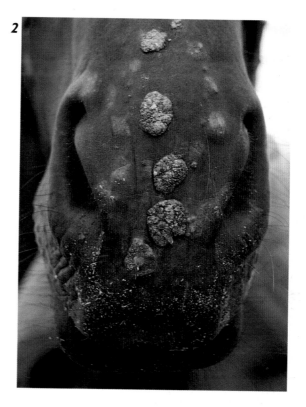

2

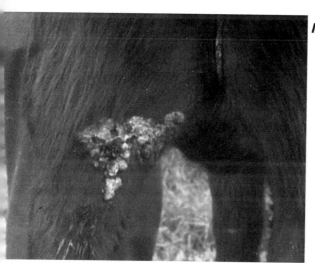

1

If the infection becomes widespread, the veterinary surgeon can send off a sample of the wart tissue and have what is called an autogenous vaccine prepared against the virus.

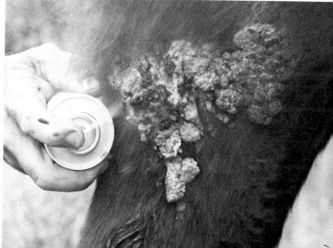

3

When the wart is persistent or in a vital area of the pony's anatomy, the veterinary surgeon may have to remove it surgically (*photo 4*).

Angleberries and warts can be ligated, and perhaps the best form of ligature is the rubber ring used with and applied by the elastrator (*photo 5*). However, when this method is used the horse must always be injected against tetanus since the wound caused by the elastrator rubber ring provides an ideal focus for the growth of the tetanus germs.

The pale flat warts seen round the nostrils and mouth of foals and yearlings often disappear spontaneously as the animal acquires a natural resistance to the causal virus.

5

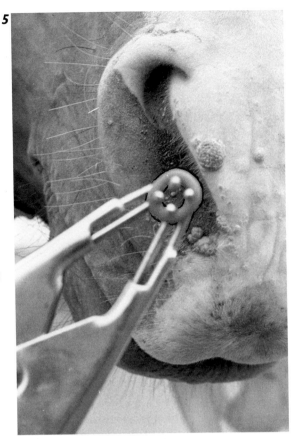

4

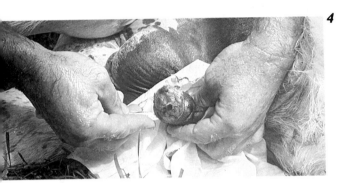

29
Sarcoids

A sarcoid (*photo 1*) is a tumour which though resembling a malignant sarcoma (i.e. a cancer) is benign and regressive. In other words it will eventually disappear, often within a matter of months. Nonetheless in the case of a large sarcoid the owner may prefer surgical removal (*photo 2*). Personally I think this should be left to the discretion of the veterinary surgeon.

1

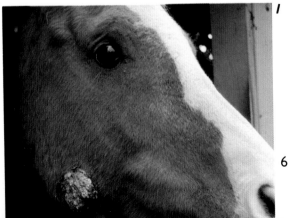

2

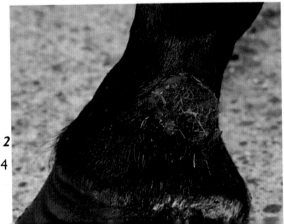

Head Region

30
The Teeth

An intelligent assessment of a horse's age can only be made by having a sound general knowledge of the teeth.

Broadly speaking, there are two types of teeth — those at the front called the incisors (*photo 1*) and those at the rear called the molars.

The portions of bare gums between the incisors and the molars are called the 'bars' and it is on these areas that the bit should rest (*photo 2*).

Horses' teeth differ from those of humans in that the horse does not chew his food — he grinds it — therefore the surfaces of the teeth are flat to allow the grinding (*photo 3*).

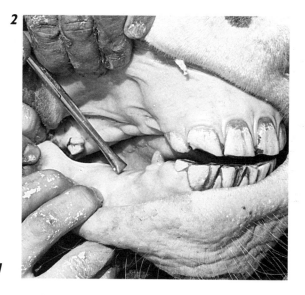

2

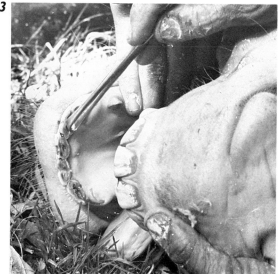

1

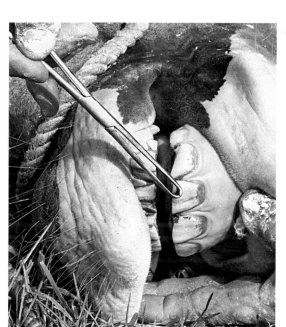

3

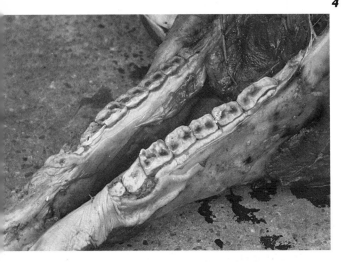

4 When a horse has all his teeth, i.e. a 'full mouth', there are six incisors on the top jaw and six incisors on the lower jaw. We describe these as two 'centrals', two 'middles' and two 'laterals'.

There are six molars on each side — top and bottom (*photo 4*).

How to tell a horse's age

When born, a foal has its two central incisors through the gum or just on the point of coming through.

The two middle incisors appear at about five weeks, and the corners at approximately eight months, so by eight months the foal has a complete set of front or incisor teeth.

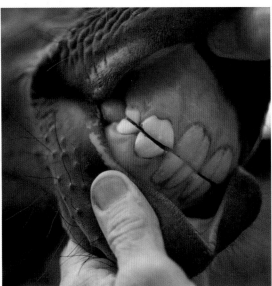

5 The front three molars on both sides are there at birth or within a fortnight.

All these teeth are temporary, or milk, teeth and are replaced, as time goes on, by the permanent teeth. The replacing is consistent and it is by the replacement of the incisor teeth that the horse's age can be accurately assessed.

The two central permanents come up through the gums at 2½ years and are in wear at 3 years (*photo 5*).

The two middle ones are up at 3½ years and are in wear at 4 years (*photo 6*).

The corners are up at 4½ years and in wear at 5 years.

All these incisor teeth have black concentric rings or cavities on their tables (*photo 7*), and it is from these that the ageing is done during the next three years.

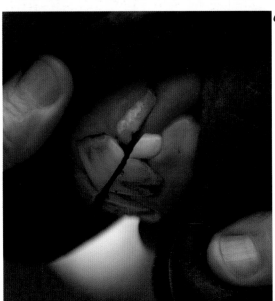

6 The cavities in the central incisors disappear at 6 years; those in the middles at 7 years and those in the corners at 8 years. At this age and thereafter a horse is said to be aged.

Estimation of age from 8 years onwards requires considerable skill and professional experience.

At 8 to 10 years a black line appears at the top of the outside of the upper corner incisor (*photo 8*). This line (the so-called 'Galvaynes groove') extends downwards with each year. It is halfway down at 15 years and it reaches the bottom of the tooth at about 20.

From 10 years onwards the incisors also start to protrude forward and the tables of the

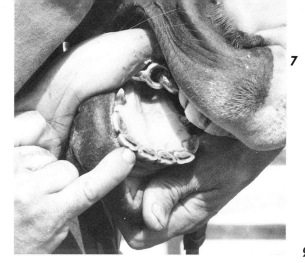

7

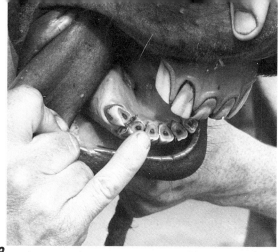

9

8

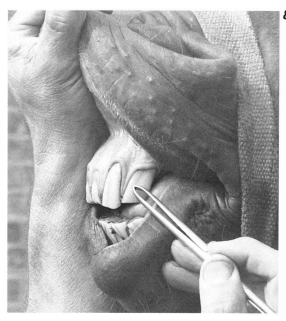

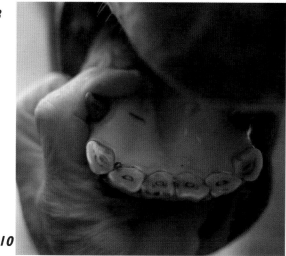

10

11

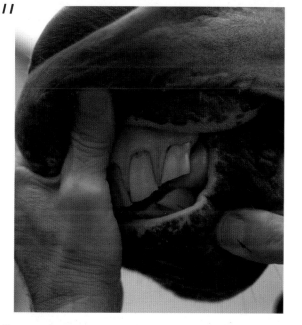

teeth, instead of being almost circular, become oval — then triangular — from front to back (*photo 9*). It is from the shape of the tables of the incisors that a veterinary surgeon of experience can tell at once whether he is dealing with an old or a young horse. It is well, therefore, for the reader to examine the photographs carefully so that he or she will be less likely to be duped. Study photo 9 and then refer back to the ovoid shape of the incisor tables in the young horse (*photo 7*).

Every knowledgeable horse owner should be able to tell at a glance whether he or she is dealing with a young or an old horse. Photo 10 shows the mouth of a 14-year-old horse, photo 11 that of a 23-year-old.

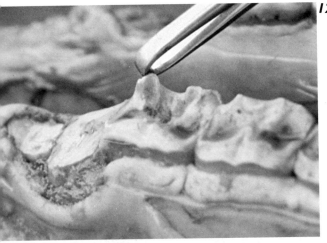

12 Care of the teeth

The horse, remember, grinds his food and thereby wears down the molar teeth. These teeth grow up out from the gums so that they always remain, or should remain, at the same level.

The tables of the lower molars slope downwards and outwards, and the tables of the upper molars slope inwards and upwards to match them.

The result of the continual grinding is that the inside edges of the lower molars may become very sharp and may scratch or cut the tongue; and the outside edges of the upper molars also become sharp and can scratch or cut the cheek (*photo 12*). In either case the horse does not eat properly and often 'quids', i.e. he drops portions of partly ground food onto the floor or ground.

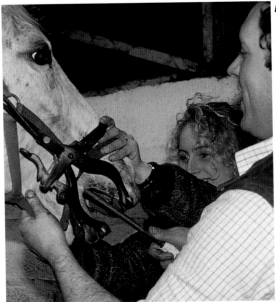

13

What to do about the teeth

The molars should be examined at least once a year by a veterinary surgeon. If there are any sharp edges or points, he will rasp them smooth (*photo 13*). This is a non-painful operation and the majority of horses will stand quietly while it is being done. The gag of choice is called the Hauseman's gag.

Sometimes, in older horses particularly, a molar may grow excessively long, usually because of a broken or shed tooth opposite. When this happens, the offending molar has to be sheared with the equine tooth shears (*photo 14*). The shears look barbaric but the operation is quite simple and absolutely painless.

14

LAMPAS

Lampas is a condition which still worries a great many horse owners. It is an oedema or dropsy of the horse's soft palate (*photo 15*), and is usually associated with the horse not eating properly; he may 'quid' and lose condition.

At one time lampas was treated by lancing the soft palate and rubbing salt into the knife wound.

Nowadays the condition is recognised as being due to a digestive disorder, and in practically every case it is seen only when the

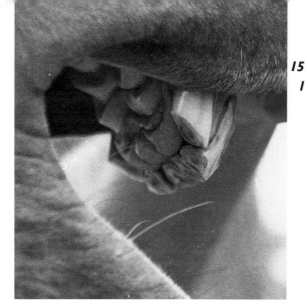

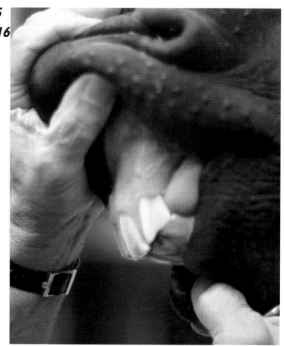

horse's teeth require attention. Almost invariably the oedema disappears after the teeth have been rasped or sheared and the horse has been given bran mashes for two or three days.

The correct treatment, therefore, is to get your veterinary surgeon to attend to the teeth immediately.

UNDERSHOT AND OVERSHOT JAWS

These are two conditions affecting the teeth and mouth that are of great importance and must not be overlooked. In an undershot jaw the teeth of the lower jaw protrude in front of those of the upper jaw. In an overshot jaw or parrot mouth (*photo 16*) the teeth of the upper jaw protrude in front of the lower jaw.

Both of these conditions are serious and constitute unsoundness. A horse suffering from either should not be purchased, as it will have difficulty in normal feeding and may find it impossible to graze.

Incidentally, it is impossible to make an accurate estimate of the animal's age if the jaw is over- or undershot.

HOW TO EXAMINE A HORSE'S MOUTH AND TEETH WITHOUT A GAG

Hold the tongue in the palm of the hand, then turn the point of the tongue upwards and backwards against the roof of the mouth and

17

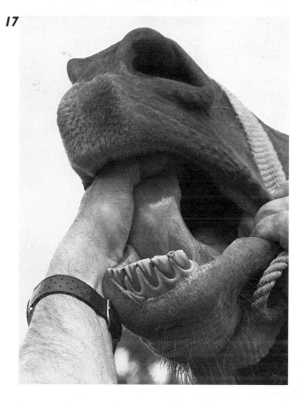

keep it there while examining the mouth either by torchlight or by feeling with the other hand (*photo 17*).

69

TOOTH EXTRACTION

Occasionally a horse gets a broken or infected tooth — usually one of the molars.

Symptoms
The patient quids and starts losing condition. A lump (*photo 18*) or fistula (*photo 19*) may develop at the side or bottom of the jaw. Careful veterinary examination of the mouth will reveal the suspect tooth. The veterinary surgeon will probably confirm the diagnosis by X-ray before operating.

Treatment
A general anaesthetic is administered (*photo 20*) and the tooth extracted (*photo 21*). Occasionally it is necessary to chisel out the offending molar, so obviously this is very much a job for the veterinary surgeon.

20

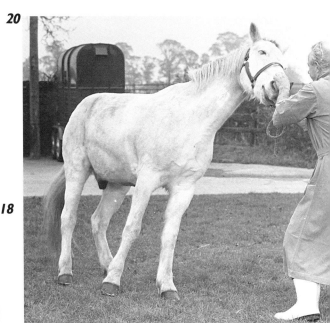

18

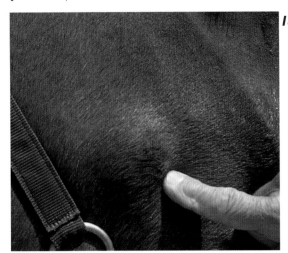

21

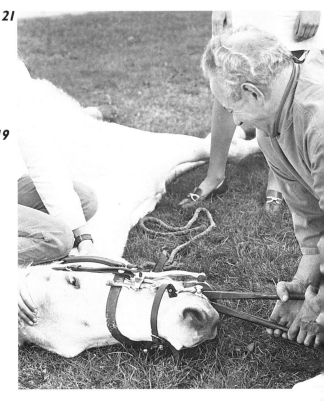

19

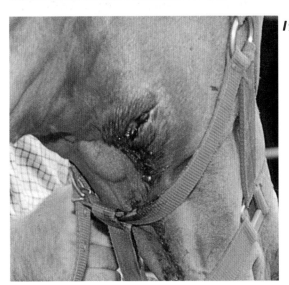

The so-called 'wolf-tooth' is present only in certain horses. It is situated in the upper jaw immediately in front of the first large premolar tooth — usually on one side only but sometimes on both.

The 'wolf-tooth' is vestigial and can be removed easily, without an anaesthetic (*photo 22*). Removal is indicated when the horse throws his head about on bit pressure or when the gum at the base is sore or inflamed.

Just occasionally the 'wolf-tooth' has a deep curved root and has to be chiselled out under a general anaesthetic.

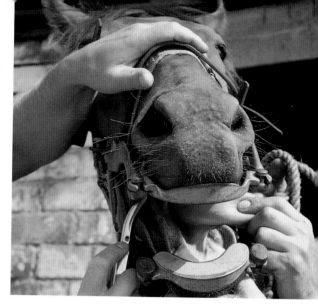

31
The Eye

Fortunately the eye in the horse is not a great source of trouble.

Simple anatomy of the eye
The eye comprises a number of distinct parts (*see diagram A*). At the front surface there is the cornea, which is a clear membrane, almost like a window with a microfine pane.

Behind the cornea is the iris. The iris dilates or contracts according to the intensity of the light it is exposed to.

To the rear of the iris there is a space containing fluid. This is called the anterior chamber.

Separating the anterior chamber from another fluid containing cavity — called the posterior chamber — is the lens. The lens can also expand and contract, being controlled by muscles which assist it to focus on near or distant objects.

The back of the eye is lined by the retina where everything the horse sees is recorded and transmitted to the brain. The horse's retina is set at an angle (*diagram B*).

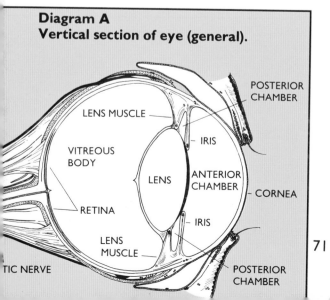

**Diagram A
Vertical section of eye (general).**

POSTERIOR CHAMBER

LENS MUSCLE

IRIS

VITREOUS BODY

LENS

ANTERIOR CHAMBER

CORNEA

RETINA

IRIS

LENS MUSCLE

OPTIC NERVE

POSTERIOR CHAMBER

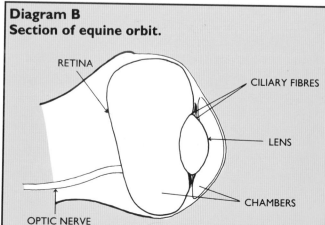

**Diagram B
Section of equine orbit.**

RETINA

CILIARY FIBRES

LENS

CHAMBERS

OPTIC NERVE

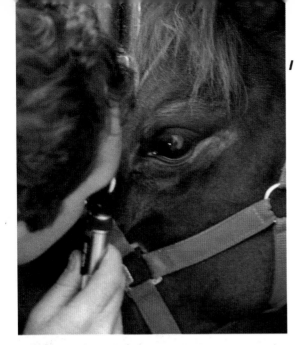

1. How to examine the eye

To do this properly, it is essential to have the horse in a completely dark box or to wait until night time. It is no use just turning the horse with his back-end to the windows; the box must be dark.

A veterinary surgeon, with an ophthalmascope, can examine the eye completely (*photo 1*), but the layman can make a very satisfactory examination without this instrument.

The routine is as follows:

Take a small pencil torch. Shine it into the eye from directly in front and then sideways (*photo 2*). In this way you can make sure that the whole surface of the cornea is absolutely clear.

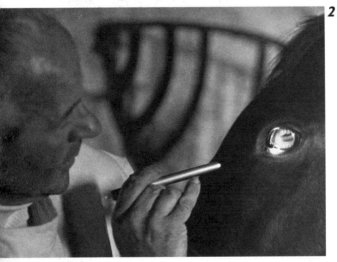

Next, shine the torch straight at the eye and watch for the iris contracting. Move the light gradually away; the iris should expand. This indicates that the animal is seeing and is reacting normally to light.

Then take a lighted candle and hold it in front of the eye (*photo 3*). You should see three images of the flame. One on the cornea — upright; one on the front of the lens — upright; and one at the back of the lens — inverted. Move the flame around and make sure that the images remain clear and distinct. This proves that both the anterior chamber and the lens are clear.

Corneal opacity (Keratitis)

Clouding of the surface of the eye is one of the commonest equine eye conditions (*photo 4*).

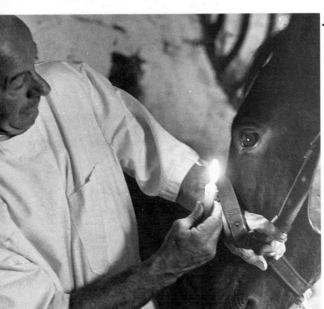

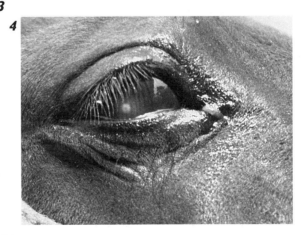

Cause

It is usually caused by an injury, perhaps being flicked by the branches of a tree or injured by a whip. There may be a puncture or a scratch on the corneal surface.

Treatment

Send for your veterinary surgeon immediately. Modern antibiotic eye dressings are extremely efficient and any delay in application can mean the loss of an eye, especially if the cornea is punctured. The antibiotic may be injected under the conjunctiva.

Prognosis

In the vast majority of cases the sight will not be lost but often a scar — a bluish-white mark shaped like a round dot or a minute whiplash — will remain permanently on the corneal surface. This constitutes an unsoundness.

Cataract

In cataract there occurs a clouding of the lens. The lens becomes grey and opaque and does not allow the light to pass through. When examining with a lighted candle, there will be no third inverted image.

Fortunately cataract is rare in the horse, though it can occasionally be congenital and can affect one or both eyes. It is a serious unsoundness.

Treatment

Surgical removal of cataracts can be performed but it does not always restore acute vision, though recent research using replacement plastic lenses bodes well for the future.

The third eyelid

On the membrana nictitans or third eyelid there occasionally grows a small tumour (*photo 5*); it is often a malignant tumour but the malignancy doesn't usually spread beyond the eye socket.

Treatment

The growth must be removed by a veterinary surgeon. The operation is simple and can be done under local anaesthesia. As a general rule it is completely successful if caught early.

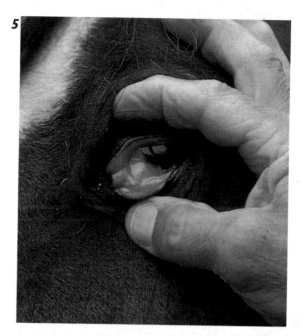

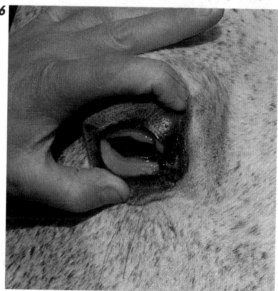

Conjunctivitis and periodic ophthalmia

Conjunctivitis or moon blindness is by far the most common condition of the horse's eye (*photo 6*).

Cause

Conjunctivitis frequently happens when the horse is at grass, particularly in warm weather. Pollen dust or other irritants get into the eye and produce an inflammation. Tears run from the affected eye and the resultant discharge attracts flies which introduce infection.

When infection starts, the eye discharge becomes 'pussy' or purulent, giving rise to the condition we call purulent conjunctivitis. The pus dries, and if the condition is not treated promptly, crusts and sores form which attract increasing numbers of flies.

If the infective agent is a leptospira (carried in rat urine and gaining entrance through a skin wound), then the much more serious recurrent condition of periodic ophthalmia may develop. With this, early diagnosis and skilled treatment are vital, otherwise blindness will result (see photo 7).

solution. Dry them thoroughly and smear the lids and around them with an antibiotic oil or ointment, either of which can be obtained from your veterinary surgeon.

If the eyes are clear, there is no need to use the saline; merely spread the antibiotic round the lids and especially in the internal canthus (or corner) (photo 8). To avoid periodic ophthalmia, use a pest controller regularly to eliminate the rat danger.

Blocked tear duct

Symptoms
A continually runny eye (photo 9).

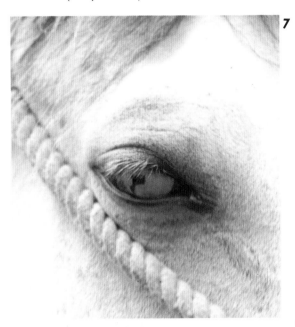

7

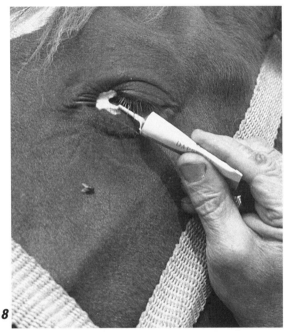

8

Treatment
Get your veterinary surgeon to diagnose the condition and prescribe treatment immediately. He may use a local dressing or inject a long-acting or broad-spectrum antibiotic under the conjunctiva and intramuscularly.

Prevention
Both conjunctivitis and periodic ophthalmia can be prevented by good management.

Bring the horse or pony up regularly when at grass. If the eyes are dirty, clean them with a piece of cotton wool soaked in warm saline

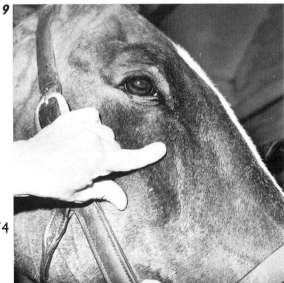

9

74

Cause

Dried discharge, hairs and debris blocking up the tear duct entrance, especially after an attack of keratitis or conjunctivitis.

Treatment

The lower opening of the duct lies just inside the nostril. Warm saline solution or antibiotic in oil syringed under pressure will clear the blockage rapidly and spectacularly (*photo 10*). Thereafter a seven to ten day course of antibiotic eye ointment is indicated to clear up any infection.

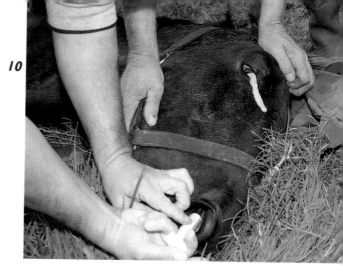

10

32
Sinuses and Sinusitis

Sinuses are to be found in the heads of all animals as well as in humans. On each side of the horse's head there are three sinuses or air spaces (*see diagram*).

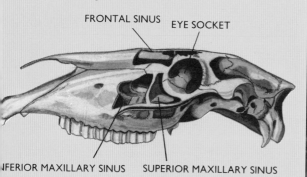

Lateral view of horse's skull with sinuses opened up.

FRONTAL SINUS   EYE SOCKET

IFERIOR MAXILLARY SINUS   SUPERIOR MAXILLARY SINUS

They are bounded on the outside by the bones that form the skull and on the inside they are separated by the nasal septum — a cartilaginous ridge running down the centre of the head from the brain.

The sinuses are lined with mucous membrane.

The top sinus is the *frontal sinus*. In the floor of this sinus there is a hole which communicates with the sinus below it — the *superior maxillary sinus*.

The superior maxillary sinus lies just below the eye on either side and each communicates with the nasal cavity.

Below this and running along the cheek is the *inferior maxillary sinus*. This sinus is largely filled by the roots of the teeth which jut up into it. As the horse or pony grows older and the teeth wear down and protrude further into the mouth, the inferior maxillary sinus becomes more of an air space.

The inferior maxillary sinus also communicates with the nasal cavity.

Sinus infection

Following a severe attack of strangles or of an ordinary cold, infection occasionally gets into these sinuses. This is indicated by pus continually dropping from one nostril (*photo 1*) or occasionally from both (*photo 2*). The pus may stream out when the horse's head is held low or when he is grazing.

Tapping on the bone with one knuckle just below the eye will often cause the horse to evince pain (*photo 3*). This confirms that the infection most commonly settles in the superior maxillary sinus.

Treatment

Treatment is a task for the veterinary surgeon only.

It consists of trephining (i.e. making a circular hole) directly into the sinus. The trephine, of course, is a special surgical instrument used only for this purpose (*photo 4*).

The trephining is generally done just below the eye into the superior maxillary sinus (*photo 5*). It is carried out usually under a local anaesthetic, with the horse standing.

It is not necessary to open into the frontal sinus, even though it may be affected, because any pus in the frontal sinus will obviously drain through into the superior maxillary sinus (*photo 6*).

The sinuses are then douched out daily through the trephine hole using a stirrup pump and a bucket of boiled water containing the correct concentration of a non-irritant antiseptic or of an antibiotic (*photo 7*).

The antiseptic or antibiotic solution swills around the frontal and superior maxillary sinus, passes through into the nasal cavity and passages and is discharged at the nostrils.

Should the infection be in the inferior maxillary sinus (*photo 8*) (possibly caused by an infected or split tooth), then this can be treated either by trephining into that sinus or by breaking down the very thin wall or septum between it and the superior maxillary sinus; and once again washing through from the original hole.

It is absolutely essential to keep the trephined hole very firmly plugged with tight cotton wool or gauze, otherwise it will heal so rapidly that, within a few days, you will be unable to get the nozzle of your syringe or pump into it.

During the period of daily douching it is an advantage to give the horse a course of antibiotic injections intramuscularly. In this way the infection is blitzed from all sides and is much more likely to clear permanently.

Some success has been claimed by the use of acupuncture.

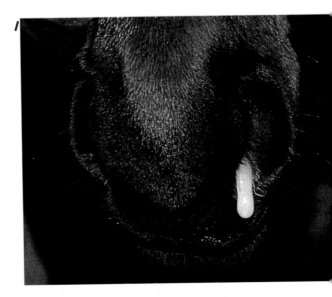

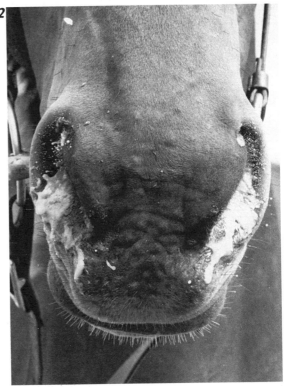

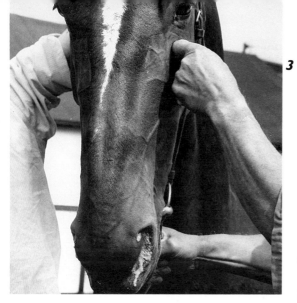

3

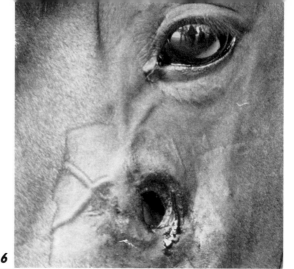

6

7

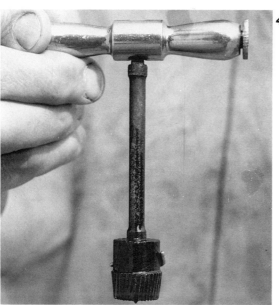

4

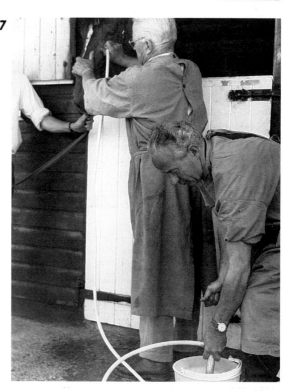

5

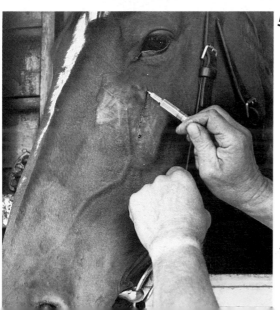

8

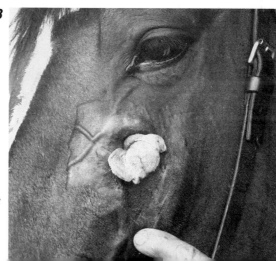

77

33
Nose Bleeding

Cause
Direct injury, chronic coughing (as in bronchitis and broken wind), growths inside the nasal chambers or a fungal infection causing ulceration of the lining of either of the gutteral pouches which extend from each side inside the throat to below the ear.

Treatment
Diagnosis and treatment are very much a matter for the veterinary surgeon. Nevertheless, a simple knowledge of first aid may save the animal.

The correct procedure is to box the horse in absolute quiet and wait for the bleeding to stop.

Never attempt to plug the nostrils with gauze or cotton wool since this may back-dam the blood into the lungs and cause a fatal mechanical pneumonia.

34
Facial Paralysis

This condition is due to an injury of the fifth trigeminal or the facial nerve which passes round the base of the ear and supplies the impulses and reflexes to the opposite side of the face.

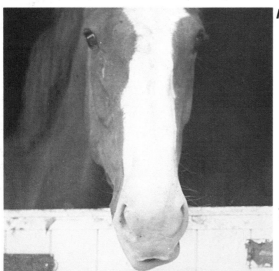

1

Symptoms
The lower lip usually droops at one side (*photo 1*). The horse may slobber when drinking.

The eye on the side opposite to the drooping lip may appear markedly smaller than the other.

Cause
Usually an injury under the horse's ear or along the side of the face.

Occasionally it arises secondary to a strangles abscess of the parotid gland, i.e. the lymph gland that lies just below the ear.

Treatment
Time and patience alone will cure facial paralysis. Local treatment is ineffective and a

78

waste of time and money.

Will it get better?
Usually, yes, though it may take up to two years to resume a normal appearance. Just occasionally the defect remains permanent but, though unsightly, it rarely, if ever, impairs the animal's usefulness.

35
Itchy Ears

Sometimes a horse or pony will show considerable irritation and distress by rubbing his ears against trees or posts and stamping his feet angrily, almost as though he has colic (*photo 1*).

Closer examination of the ears may reveal a black waxy discharge. The horse or pony strongly resents the ears being touched. In the summer flies, attracted by the smell of the discharge, will be massed around the ears and will give the pony no rest.

Cause
Not fully established but thought to be a mite similar to the one involved in the itchy tail. Swabs can be taken from the ear contents and examined microscopically (*photo 2*).

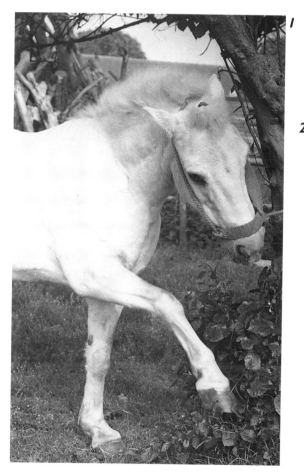

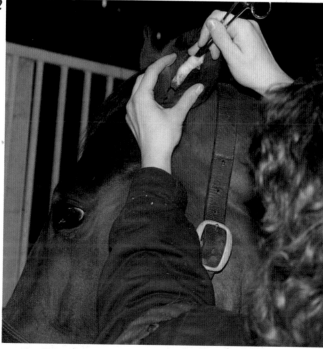

Treatment

Again, a job for your veterinary surgeon. He will probably dress the ears with a benzyl benzoate dressing or certainly one containing an active ingredient against mites (benzene hexachloride is a favourite drug prescribed) (*photo 3*). The ears will require three dressings at intervals of five to seven days.

Keep the patient inside during the day as a protection against the flies. This common sense precaution will help considerably in clearing the condition quickly.

Prevention

The best prevention is prompt veterinary treatment at first sight. Remember, itchy ears can be kept under control, and the sooner treatment is started the better it is for both the patient and the veterinary surgeon.

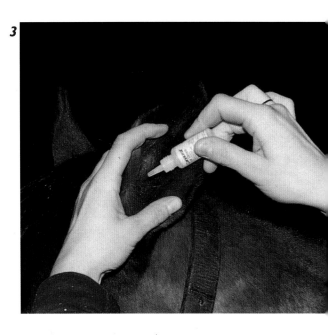

3

36
Headshaking

This becomes a problem when the horse shakes its head for no apparent reason (*photo 1*), especially when the shaking is so severe that it makes riding difficult or even dangerous.

1

Symptoms

The headshaking is usually seen at exercise, especially at the trot, and it often manifests itself after five or ten minutes with the head being violently thrown upwards and downwards and accompanied by snorting or sneezing. Less frequently the head is thrown from side to side and just occasionally in circles. If the exercise is continued the tendency is for the shaking to get progressively worse and often for the horse to attempt rubbing its nose on its foreleg or on the ground.

Cause

Since the symptoms most often appear in warm sunny weather and in the country, it is feasible that the commonest cause is an allergy similar to hay fever in humans, though not just an allergy to grass pollen but to those pollens associated with trees, hedgerows and even a crop of rape.

Certain cases are due to more apparent causes like mouth or tongue wounds, ear mites, sinusitis, fibrositis or eye disease, but these occur independent of exercise and environment and can usually be diagnosed by a veterinary surgeon.

Treatment
Treatment depends entirely on the diagnosis and is never easy or straightforward. It's very much a job for the veterinary surgeon, who may have to resort to surgery or acupuncture.

37
Poll Evil and Fistulous Withers

Poll evil and fistulous withers occur when the bursa at the top of the poll, or the one at the height of the withers, becomes inflamed (*photo 1*).

Cause
Usually an injury.

Symptoms
A well marked swelling which may or may not be painful to the touch (*photo 2*). The painful ones usually increase in size until they burst. When this happens a permanent running sore (a fistula) often develops (*photo 3*). The reason for this is that occasionally a germ (the cattle abortion germ, *Brucella abortus*, in fact) is present in these two bursae and the bug starts

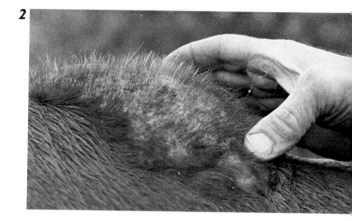

2

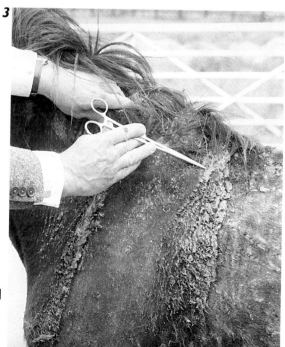

3

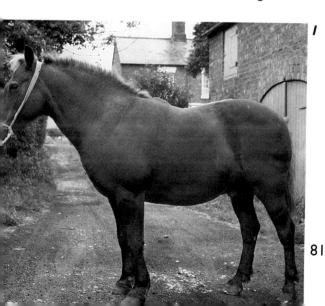

1

to multiply as soon as the inflammation commences. It continues to multiply — producing heat, pain and often death of neighbouring tissues — until the wall of the bursa gives way. Other bacteria may be involved.

Treatment

If the condition is spotted early, one or several injections of cattle abortion vaccine will very often cause the inflammation to subside.

If it does not and a fistula develops, then often the only answer is radical surgery in which the bursa together with any surrounding damaged tissue is dissected right out.

If the swelling remains soft, fluctuating and painless, then it can be disregarded though it may be necessary to have special alterations made to the saddle or the poll piece of the head collar and bridle.

Obviously the decision as to which treatment should be employed must be left to your veterinary surgeon.

Brucellosis affecting other parts of the horse

Very occasionally when horses are grazed in the same field as cattle heavily infected with brucellosis, they can develop obscure lamenesses involving leg bursae and tendon sheaths. *Brucella abortus* is involved in these cases, but the diagnosis is very difficult and should always be left to a veterinary surgeon.

Fortunately, brucellosis has now been virtually eradicated in Britain.

Upper Respiratory Tract and Thorax or Chest

38
The Common Cold

In the horse the common cold is very similar to that in man.

Cause
It is caused by a virus and, as in humans, there are various strains of the horse cold virus.

Symptoms
Similar to those in humans. There is lassitude, inappetence, shivering, a rise in temperature to 103°F or 104°F (39.4°C or 40°C) and an increased pulse rate to around 50 or 60. Usually a muco-purulent discharge develops, but the glands are not affected.

Treatment
The important thing to remember is that the equine cold, like the human one, is highly contagious and can rapidly spread through an entire stable. The first essential in treatment, therefore, is complete isolation.

Thereafter concentrate on commonsense good nursing. Rug the horse up and bandage the legs (the extremities particularly get very cold) (*photo 1*). Allow plenty of fresh air but

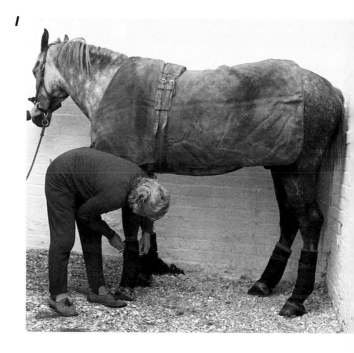

no draughts.

Put the patient on a light diet of bran mashes and hay.

Your veterinary surgeon will probably prescribe an electuary containing a febrifuge and a course of antibiotic injections to prevent secondary infection. As in humans the patient often develops a sore throat and a nasty cough, and undoubtedly a suitable electuary smeared on the tongue two or three times a day has a soothing effect (*photo 2*). Some owners regard the electuary as old fashioned, but many of the older treatments have much to recommend them. It is my experience that the best results are obtained by combining the old with the new.

3

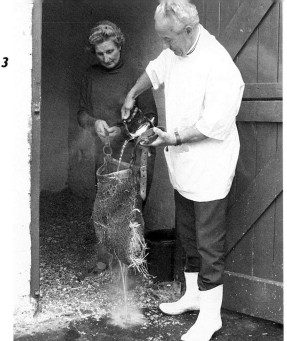

2

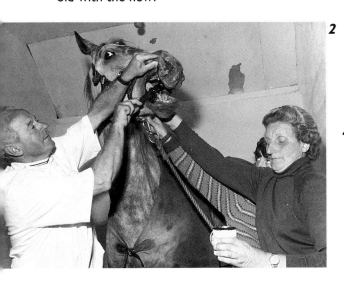

As the case develops, the nasal catarrh usually appears. If this is causing distress, the horse should be 'steamed' twice daily. 'Steaming' is done by using an old feed bag with lots of holes in it, low down, to allow the entrance of air. Put some hay in the bottom of the bag and sprinkle it over with friar's balsam or oil of eucalyptus. Pour boiling water over the medicated hay and a powerfully smelling steam will rise up (*photo 3*). Stick the patient's head in the bag; he will reluctantly inhale the medicated steam but when he does, the catarrhal discharge will flow freely and do a great deal towards clearing his head (*photo 4*). During steaming it is wise to stand by all the time in case the horse should panic or get into any difficulties.

Twice daily, close all the windows. Remove all rugs and bandages, groom the patient all over (*photo 5*), then replace them.

4

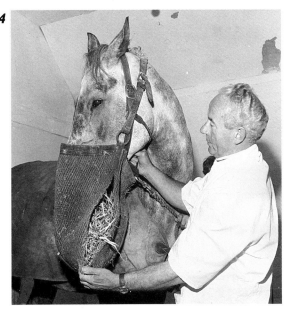

5

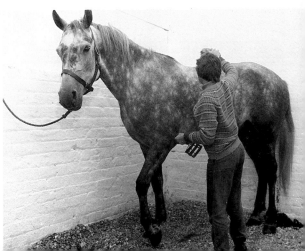

This has much the same refreshing effect on the horse as a bath does to a bed-ridden patient and in my experience it forms a very important part of successful treatment. After all, it is only commonsense.

How long does recovery take?

The average case of cold will run its course in about ten days. This means that the horse has to be nursed and rested for at least a fortnight. After that time, of course, he must be started only with gentle exercise and brought into full work gradually over a period of another week or ten days.

Occasionally — and this is very important —

the cough may hang on for months. This does not necessarily mean that the horse is broken-winded but, so long as the cough persists, the horse should not be worked. The same thing may happen after a severe attack of strangles (see page 86). In both the common cold and strangles, there may develop a severe pharyngitis and laryngitis, and it is these conditions which sometimes take a long time to clear. In fact the pharyngitis and laryngitis may become so severe that an emergency tracheotomy (see tubing a horse, page 95) may be necessary to enable the patient to breathe freely during the convalescent period.

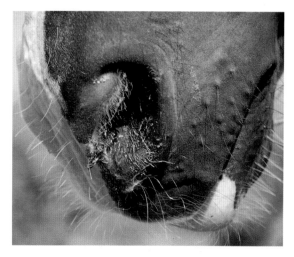

Typical nasal discharge of the common cold.

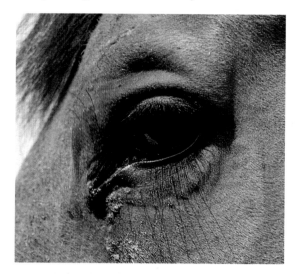

Typical eye of the common cold.

Conjunctivitis secondary to the cold.

Treating conjunctivitis with long-acting antibiotic.

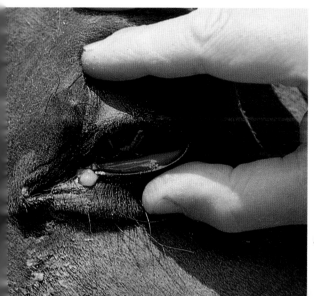

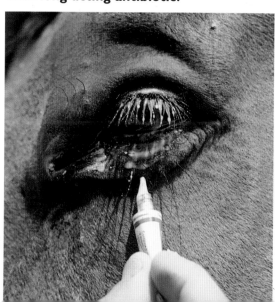

39
Strangles

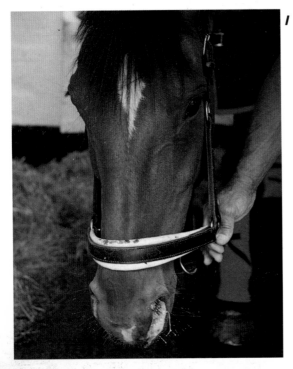

1 Strangles is caused by a pus-forming organism called the *Streptococcus equi*. It is an infectious and a highly contagious disease which can spread like wild-fire through a stable or at pasture.

Symptoms

The early symptoms are similar to those of the common cold, viz. lassitude, inappetence, elevated temperature, and increased pulse. However, in strangles the nasal discharge appears rapidly and this very quickly becomes purulent — thick wads of pus running from the nostrils (*photo 1*).

There is invariably a sore throat and the horse may have difficulty in swallowing.

Within a few hours the lymphatic glands of the head start to swell (*photo 2*). The lymph glands most commonly affected are those between the angles of the lower jaw, but the parotid glands behind and underneath the ears may also be affected.

The glands swell up, are very painful to the touch, and eventually abscesses form.

2 On a few occasions other lymphatic glands in different parts of the body become affected; when this happens the condition is known as 'bastard strangles'.

Treatment

The same principles of nursing outlined for treatment of the common cold should be rigorously adhered to, but with strangles isolation must be absolute and complete. In addition, all feeding and grooming utensils must be disinfected twice daily (*photo 3*), and any bedding removed from the box or stall should be burned.

Soft, moist mashes (*photo 4*) are even more

86

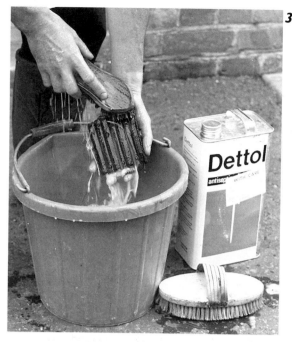

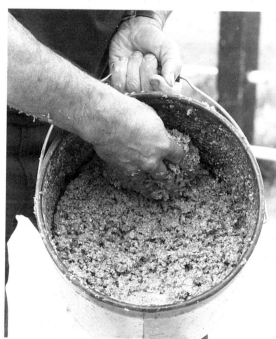

3 hot water containing epsom salts (one tablespoonful to the gallon) twice daily. This will bring the abscess to a head ready for your veterinary surgeon to lance (*photo 5*). You can tell when the abscess is ready by feeling with the point of your finger — a distinct soft point should be present. Needless to say, rapid relief to the patient follows the lancing and the draining of the pus.

In the vast majority of cases the strangles abscesses are confined to the head, but occasionally in 'bastard strangles' they may appear on any part of the body where there is a lymph node — the inside or outside of the legs or internally in the mesenteric glands, the liver, kidneys, etc. In the odd case where this does occur the horse may die or have to be slaughtered. Fortunately the modern use of antibiotics has made the fatal case of strangles a rarity.

A course of antibiotics is therefore vital, and it is important to start the course as early as possible — at the first sign of symptoms — especially if strangles is known to be in the area.

4

Prevention
Strangles vaccines are available. These vary in their efficiency in different parts of the world and, like all vaccines, require fourteen days to produce their effect.

5
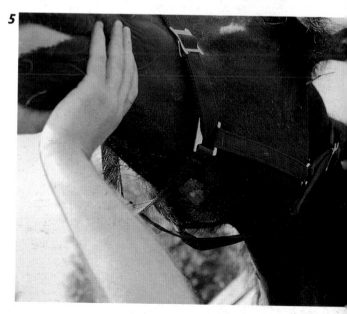

important than in the common cold because of the inevitable sore throat. Steaming, too, is vital in strangles cases and should be done conscientiously at least twice daily. After each spell wash the nostrils and smear with vaseline.

The swollen glands should be fomented with

40
Equine Influenza (The Cough)

This condition has been such a nuisance in the horse world during recent years that I think it best to deal with it on a simple question-and-answer basis.

What causes it?
The cough (*photo 1*) is caused by a virus — a myxovirus. This is related to the human influenza virus, type A.

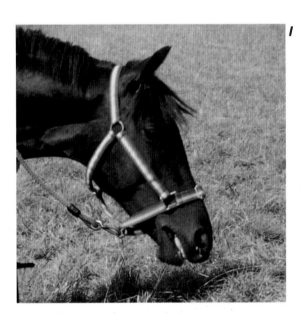

Where does it occur?
Equine influenza occurs all over the world, and has been known in Britain for many years.

When is it most likely to occur?
The cough is much worse some years than others. It is especially common during hot dry summers, and from July to September.

At what age does it attack?
All ages can be affected, but young foals are particularly susceptible.

Is it infectious?
Highly so. It sweeps through stables and studs; spreads rapidly throughout an entire district; and can affect 90-100 per cent of the horses, ponies and foals.

How serious is it?
It is rarely fatal in adults unless untreated complications are allowed to develop. In foals, however, mortality may be high.

Where does the virus strike?
The virus causes an inflammation of the linings of the bronchioles, i.e. the small air spaces of the lungs. This explains why the typical case of influenza does not develop a pussy nasal discharge, only a slight colourless or watery discharge from the nostrils.

How long does it take to develop?
The incubation period is very short — a few days only.

What are the symptoms?
There is an initial fever which rapidly subsides and is often unnoticed. Then the coughing starts and this is really the only important symptom.

The cough, initially moist, quickly gets harsh, dry and painful, and many horses become markedly distressed. The coughing persists with little or no clear nasal discharge; neither the eyes nor the glands are involved. The discharge may become purulent.

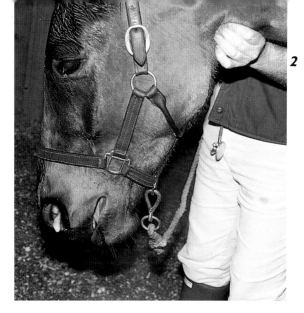

Is there any treatment?

Sensible nursing is the main therapy. Stop working the patient immediately and do not start again until the cough has disappeared. This may mean a rest of from several weeks to, occasionally, even several months. Consult your veterinary surgeon immediately regarding the protection of any young susceptible foals.

If the patient should stop eating or appear fevered (*photo 2*), your veterinary surgeon

2 will prescribe a course of antibiotic injections to control any secondary pneumonia organisms. Failure to do this can be fatal.

If the horse is eating normally and the weather is favourable, turn it out to grass until the cough disappears.

Can it be prevented?

Highly efficient vaccines giving simultaneous protection against tetanus are available.

Two doses of the vaccine are given intramuscularly at an interval of six weeks. Thereafter full protection is given by a single booster dose once a year.

There is no site reaction and the vaccine can be used safely in the pregnant mare up to eight months. The dose is only 1 cc, and a full 12 months' immunity is given.

Unfortunately, foals under three months cannot be vaccinated, but if the mothers have been protected, a fair degree of immunity is passed onto the foal through the colostrum or first milk.

Best time of year to vaccinate?

Breeding mares — October or November. Other animals — March or April.

41
Equine Rhinopneumonitis (Equine Herpes)

Another respiratory condition recently diagnosed by research scientists has been given the rather complicated name of equine rhinopneumonitis.

Cause

The equine herpes virus type number 1 referred to by researchers as EHV-1.

The virus is highly contagious and has become a source of increasing trouble especially in pedigree studs and racing stables.

Symptoms

The virus settles in the mucous membranes (linings) of the respiratory system where it quickly produces an elevated temperature, inappetence, a nasty nasal discharge, coughing and depression.

The lowered resistance thus produced may allow secondary bacteria to move in to produce a serious bronchopneumonia — hence the name rhinopneumonitis.

The virus is especially dangerous in studs,

since it can produce abortion and mare death in some cases (*photo 1*).

Treatment
The same as for the other respiratory problems. Isolation and careful nursing with antibiotics being used only to prevent or treat secondary infection. Obviously brood mares require special veterinary supervision.

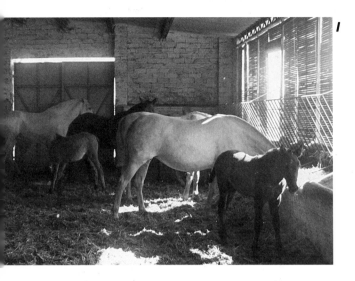

1

Prevention
A vaccine with the proprietary name Rhinomune is available. It is given intramuscularly with an initial course of two injections at four to eight week intervals followed by a single annual booster.

Although in-foal mares can be vaccinated at two and five months of pregnancy, Rhinomune does not prevent abortion. However another proprietary product called Pneumabort offers considerable protection against abortion and can be used in conjunction with Rhinomune. No doubt research will continue and improved combined vaccines will be forthcoming. This is vitally essential since there is at least one other equine herpes virus (subtype 2) and the available vaccines have yet to prove effective against this.

42
Pneumonia

The term 'pneumonia' simply means lack of air. In the horse, as in all other animals and in humans, this condition is brought about by inflammation of the lungs.

Cause
Infection by a virus or bacteria.

Mechanical pneumonias can be caused either by direct injury or by fluid finding its way into the lungs during drenching.

Symptoms
In the virus or bacterial pneumonia the infection usually starts in the lower part of *one* or *both* lungs, giving rise respectively to what we call 'single' or 'double' pneumonia. The infection spreads from the bottom lobes upwards (*see diagram*).

As in all other inflammations, there occurs

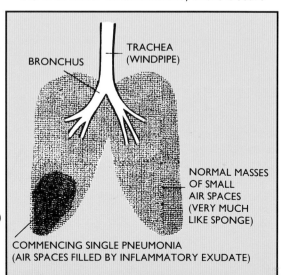

BRONCHUS

TRACHEA (WINDPIPE)

NORMAL MASSES OF SMALL AIR SPACES (VERY MUCH LIKE SPONGE)

COMMENCING SINGLE PNEUMONIA (AIR SPACES FILLED BY INFLAMMATORY EXUDATE)

an initial swelling and this blocks up the air spaces which would normally take in the air and oxygen. The swelling is followed by an inflammatory exudation and this closes up still more of the lung spaces. There is a persistent high temperature.

Breathing becomes painful and difficult, producing coughing and the typical pneumonic rapid shallow respirations.

If large parts of both lungs become affected, the horse is unable to take in sufficient oxygen to keep its heart and body going and death will follow.

Treatment
Immediate skilled veterinary attention is vital since a prolonged course of a broad-spectrum antibiotic will be necessary to effect a cure.

Of course, as in the common cold and in all other respiratory infections, good nursing is extremely important (see page 83). In fact it is absolutely vital.

43
Hypostatic Pneumonia

Hypostatic pneumonia occurs when a horse is unable to rise and lies flat out on its side for any length of time. This type of pneumonia is caused by an accumulation of blood and blood serum at the base of the horse's lungs.

Prevention
Get the veterinary surgeon to raise the horse onto its legs as soon as possible. He will probably use a long thick rope, a tripod (or beam if the horse is inside) and a set of pulley blocks. The horse can then be put in slings and the veterinary surgeon can proceed to treat the cause of the recumbency.

Until this can be done the patient must be turned from one side to the other at hourly intervals.

Hypostatic pneumonia is one of the main reasons why a neglected recumbent horse rarely lives for any length of time.

44
Pleurisy

The word 'pleurisy' simply means an inflammation of the pleura, i.e. the fine membrane that lines the chest and covers the lungs. The inflammation is caused by bacteria.

Pleurisy rarely happens on its own. It occurs along with or as a sequel to colds, pneumonia or strangles.

In the early stages the pleurisy is usually a 'dry' pleurisy, i.e. there is no exudate or fluid between the two layers of the pleura: both surfaces (the inside of the part lining the chest wall and the outside of that covering the lung) are inflamed and roughened. Obviously there is considerable pain as the two rough surfaces rub together during breathing.

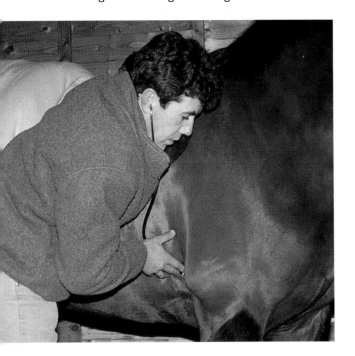

Symptoms

Breathing is shallow and rapid, and careful examination of the chest with a stethoscope (*photo 1*) reveals the dry rough sounds similar in some ways to two pieces of sand paper being rubbed together. This, of course, is a job for your veterinary surgeon.

As the case advances, fluid is discharged into the pleural cavity. The pleurisy is now described as a 'wet' pleurisy and an experienced veterinary surgeon will have little difficulty in diagnosing this stage.

Treatment

The veterinary surgeon will prescribe antibiotic therapy. If the pleural exudate is excessive, the horse will have difficulty in breathing and it may be necessary to 'tap the fluid off'. Puncture is effected, with a thin trocar and cannula, behind the elbow. In some cases several gallons of fluid may have to be drained off. If this is not done, the fluid may cause asphyxia or suffocation by simple pressure on the outside surfaces of the lungs — a pressure which prevents the intake of sufficient air or oxygen.

45
The Horse's Wind

When a horse is sold it is frequently warranted 'sound in wind'. This means that the horse's breathing apparatus is in perfect working order.

A sound horse breathes inwards and outwards through its nostrils, *never* through its mouth.

The air travels up the nasal passages into the larynx or voice box, through the trachea and into the lungs, one on either side of the chest.

The lungs can be likened to two sponges, i.e. they are made up of innumerable minute cavities or spaces all connecting one with the other (*see diagram A*).

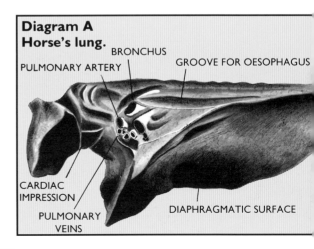

Diagram A
Horse's lung.

BRONCHUS

PULMONARY ARTERY

GROOVE FOR OESOPHAGUS

CARDIAC IMPRESSION

PULMONARY VEINS

DIAPHRAGMATIC SURFACE

In these cavities the air, when it fills them, exchanges its oxygen for carbon dioxide which has been brought there by the blood. The blood is revitalised by this essential oxygen.

The oxygenated blood then travels throughout the body to all the muscles and tissues where it gives up its oxygen to provide heat and energy, and takes in the carbon dioxide.

Obviously the harder a horse works, the more oxygen it requires. When a horse is galloped, its breathing is accelerated and the heart rate rises, i.e. the blood is being pumped faster and faster round the circular course to get more and more oxygen to the muscles where the extra energy is required.

'High blowing'

When a horse starts to move, you frequently hear a distinct purring noise on expiration, i.e. when the horse breathes out. This noise is known as 'high blowing' and is caused by a flapping of the false nostril inside the other nostril. It is *not* an unsoundness.

'Bridle noise'

Where a keen horse is being held in with his head pulled into his chest and his neck arched, you may get another expiratory sound rather like roaring but not so pronounced (*photo 1*).

This is a 'bridle noise' — a whistling noise on expiration. Like high blowing, a bridle noise is not an unsoundness.

In fact, both high blowing and bridle noises are minor things which pass off quickly as soon as the horse is put into work and his head and neck are allowed to move freely.

Broken wind

If the minute cavities in the lungs tear so that one small hole joins with its neighbour or neighbours, comparatively large spaces may form. When this happens the condition is called emphysema: if this becomes at all extensive, the horse is 'broken winded'.

Because of the emphysematous spaces, the normal inspiration does not bring in sufficient air to provide the oxygen required nor does it take away all the carbon dioxide. It is therefore necessary for the broken-winded horse to take two inspiratory gasps to fully fill its lungs, and the effort, especially if the horse is at work, results in a very nasty chronic cough (*photo 2*), often described as a 'deep sepulchral cough'. For the same reason expiration takes place in two stages.

2

1

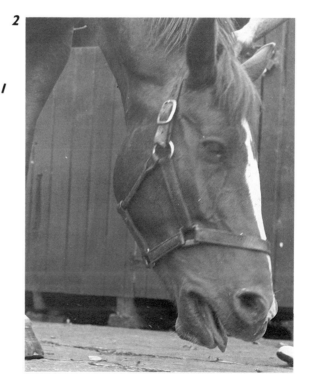

Symptoms

The condition is first diagnosed by the characteristic deep cough which is present even at rest and is often most marked when he is feeding. And secondly, by the double expiration which can be seen by looking carefully at his flanks where the double expiratory lift produces a pronounced furrow or groove — the so-called 'broken-winded furrow' (*photo 3*).

Treatment

There is no treatment for broken wind, but the cough is considerably alleviated if all the food, including the hay, is damped to keep down the dust (*photo 4*). For the same reason, peat moss should not be used for bedding. The ideal bedding for a broken-winded horse (including those suffering from dust allergies, page 98) is sand, sawdust or wood shavings. Shredded paper, now available in bales, is also ideal.

It is probably better, however, to keep a broken-winded horse out at grass throughout the year. In this way, a mild case may remain fit for slow gentle exercise for some time.

If he has to be kept in, pelleted food is preferable to hay.

4

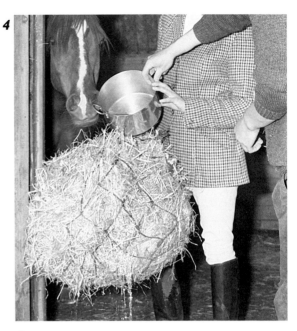

Roaring

In the larynx or voice box there are two flaps — one on either side as illustrated (*diagram B*) — which normally move backwards and forwards as the horse breathes. The flaps are like two small swing doors.

The nerves that supply these doors sometimes become paralysed, particularly on the left side. The result is that the improperly controlled flap lies partly or completely across the larynx and interferes with the passage of the air being drawn into the lungs. This

3

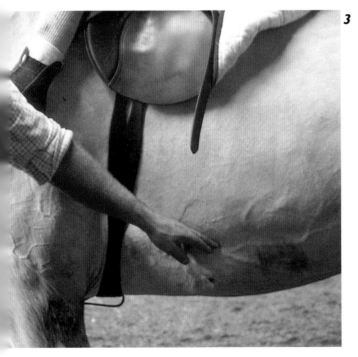

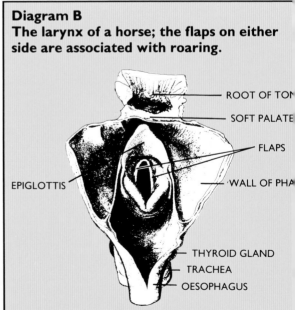

Diagram B
The larynx of a horse; the flaps on either side are associated with roaring.

ROOT OF TON

SOFT PALATE

FLAPS

EPIGLOTTIS

WALL OF PHA

THYROID GLAND

TRACHEA

OESOPHAGUS

produces a sound varying from a whistle to a marked roaring noise. It occurs, however, on **inspiration**, not on expiration.

The diagnosis is confirmed by the use of an endoscope (*photo 5*).

Is roaring an unsoundness?

It is a definite unsoundness because the obstruction or obstructions stop the air getting into the lungs and the horse soon becomes breathless when hunted. In fact, often the roarer has to be pulled up and rested periodically.

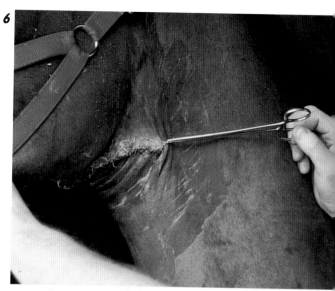

6

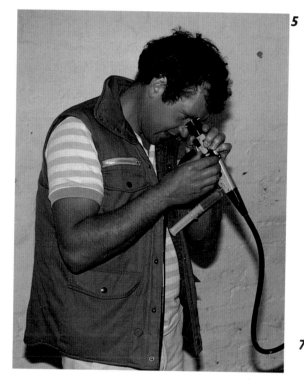

5

Treatment

Roaring is incurable by ordinary treatments, but the condition can be partially or completely cured by a surgical procedure called Hobday's Operation (*photo 6*). With luck a successful job may make the horse perfectly serviceable for hunting or even for racing. In racehorses, however, many people prefer 'tubing'.

Tubing a horse

Tubing a horse means surgically inserting a

special tracheotomy tube into the horse's windpipe (*photo 7*). The operation should be performed only by a veterinary surgeon and always under a suitable anaesthetic.

When should a horse be tubed?

A horse can be tubed if he is a roarer and if the surgical roaring operation has not been performed.

He can be tubed at any time where there is marked difficulty in breathing, e.g. during an acute strangles or a sudden acute attack of urticaria.

The technique of operation is very much a matter for the veterinary surgeon.

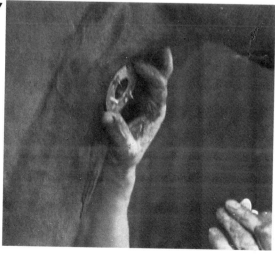

7

46
How to Test a Horse's Wind

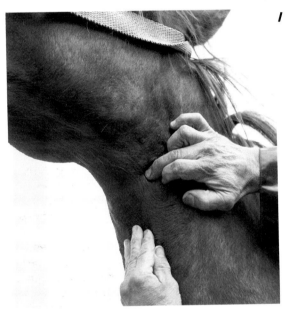

The following routine has been evolved from a lifetime's experience of examining horses:

1. Check for scars over the windpipe (*photo 1*), and make sure that the skin is free over the larynx or voice box.

2. Watch the horse quietly at rest in his box; look carefully at his flank for any double lift.

3. Listen intently, with the ear or with a stethoscope (*photo 2*) to both lungs for any emphysematous noises. Obviously this has to be done by a veterinary surgeon. Emphysematous noises can be described as similar to those made by blowing over the top of an empty bottle.

4. Squeeze the horse's larynx with the thumb and fore-finger (*photo 3*). If he coughs be suspicious.

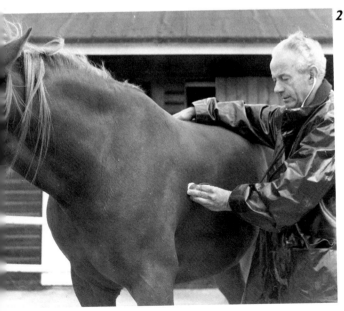

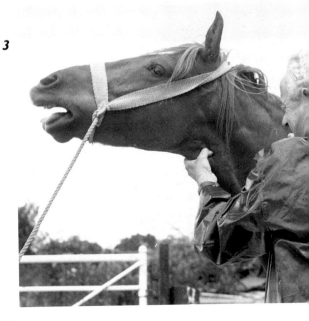

4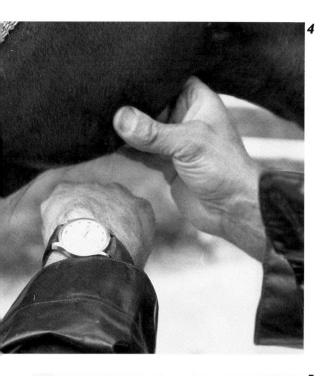

5. Check his pulse and temperature* (*photos 4 & 5*). These should be normal; if elevated, then the cough could be due to a common cold or to some other infection. If the temperature and/or pulse are in any way abnormal, the horse should not be tested further until he has completely recovered.

6. If the pulse and temperature are normal, then put on the saddle and bridle and take him out into the field.

Canter the horse in a small circle on the right rein, or if someone else is riding, stand at the **outside** of the circle so that the horse passes very close and his breathing is clearly audible. Make him do several circles at a slow hack canter. Then put him onto the other rein and repeat the circling.

7. If no suspicious noise or distress is spotted, send him on a sharp gallop across the field — fast — for a distance of at least half a mile. When he is pulled up, listen very carefully at his nostrils for any sign of whistling or roaring which, remember, will be **heard on**

5 **inspiration**. Also take another look at his flanks and check again for the double lift. If a veterinary surgeon — listen again to the lungs for emphysema.

8. One final point. Always beware when a horse is brought up from grass with a big belly and carrying excess weight ('pig fat'). Often such animals may make noises similar to whistling or roaring. It is much better to go back at a later date to see such a horse when he is fit or fined down, otherwise you may wrongly condemn him.

Grunting to the stick

The idea behind testing the horse by prodding its flank sharply with a stick is that it frightens the animal. The sudden fear makes the horse shut its glottis and blow out. If the larynx is normal, there should be no noise. An abnormal larynx which doesn't close properly produces a noise or a grunt.

Although a valuable aid to diagnosis, the grunting in itself is not conclusive proof of unsoundness.

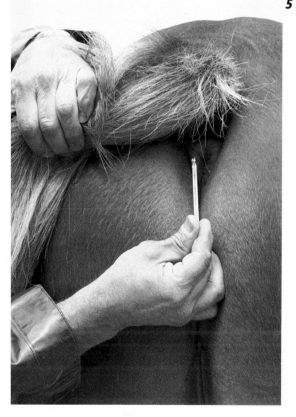

* For normal pulse and respiration, see page 3.

47
Thyroid Enlargement (Goitre)

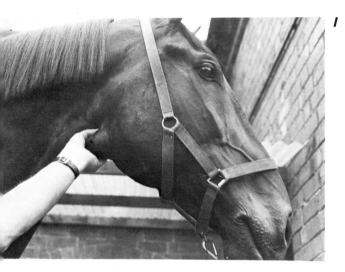

1 The thyroid gland, consisting of two lobes and a connecting branch, is situated closely in connection with the upper end of the trachea or windpipe (*photo 1*).

Just occasionally, if this gland is not functioning properly, it increases in size. When this happens, pressure on the windpipe can cause marked inspiratory and expiratory noises.

Treatment comprises the daily administration of minute quantities of iodine in the food. Your veterinary surgeon will advise and prescribe the correct dosage.

I know of one client who cured such a case by feeding a tablespoonful of iodised budgerigar seed daily in the horse's feed.

48
Dust Allergies

In my experience horses with so-called 'dust allergies' are in fact broken-winded cases with distinct emphysema in one or both lungs. The condition is often described as 'heaves' or asthma and treatment is exactly as prescribed for broken wind.

The allergies are not caused by the dust alone but by spores of a mould or fungus attached to the dust. These spores are present in large quantities in hay and straw, especially if badly made. This means that all traditional stables and boxes are potentially dangerous.

Fortunately, however, only a small percentage of horses are sensitive to the spores. When they are, the resultant allergy causes the small air spaces in the lungs to become blocked with discharges and the subsequent persistent coughing produces the emphysema and broken wind.

The obvious and only answer with these cases is to stable as little as possible, to feed with warm bran mashes plus a complete pelleted food, and if you have to stable, to eliminate all sources of the spores by bedding on sand, sawdust or shavings.

Shredded paper, supplied in bales, has proved ideal bedding for all such cases (*photo 1*).

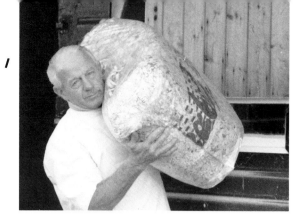

1

49
African Horse Sickness

Although this disease has so far not appeared in Britain, America or most of Europe, a comparatively recent severe outbreak in Spain plus a flare up in Portugal warrants its inclusion here.

Cause
A virus called *Reoviridae.*

Predisposing causes
Warm low-lying swampy environments such as valleys and river estuaries.

Method of spread
Transmitted by a natural biting gnat which is most active during the hot summer months.

Animals affected
Mainly horses. Mules and donkeys less frequently.

It is important to note that the virus can also enter the human eye directly from an infected atmosphere.

Symptoms
An initial very high fever with swelling around the head and neck. This is followed by coughing and conjunctivitis and later a filthy evil-smelling nasal discharge.

The swelling spreads to the abdomen and eventually floods the lungs, causing asphyxiation. Peculiarly enough the animal often continues to eat until a few hours before death.

Treatment
There is none.

Prevention
Vaccination two months prior to the danger period plus control of the insects. Obviously susceptible animals should be housed at night.

Oesophagus and Abdomen

50
Choke

One of the most serious conditions met with in horses, and certainly one of the most difficult to treat, is 'choke', i.e. when the horse's oesophagus gets blocked up anywhere between the pharynx (throat) and stomach.

Cause
Occasionally an apple or potato gets stuck just behind the epiglottis, but it is my experience that most cases of choke are caused by dry bran (*photo 1*) or dry beet pulp.

Symptoms
The patient is in some distress. He coughs, slobbers and may appear to vomit with the resultant discharge running from the nostrils as well as from the mouth (*photo 2*).

Usually the choked horse refuses all food or

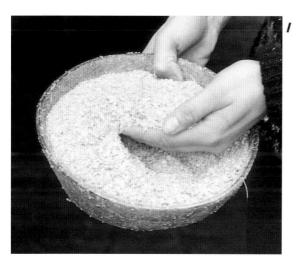

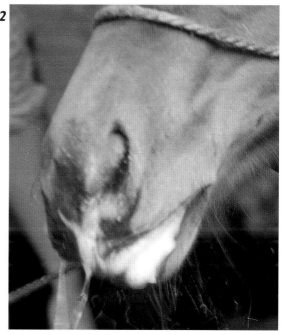

water, though occasionally if the lower part of the oesophagus is involved, he may swallow some water only to cough it up again almost immediately.

Treatment
Definitely a job for your veterinary surgeon. He will probably hospitalise the patient and keep him under constant observation. Daily injections of carbachol (carbamylcholine chloride) and muscle relaxants may be required for up to a week or even longer. Several first-class muscle relaxants are now available to veterinary surgeons.

Prevention
Never let your horse or pony graze in an orchard during the apple season. Never feed potatoes and never, under any circumstances, feed dry bran or dry beet pulp.

51
Colic

Colic is the name given to a symptom, namely abdominal pain. According to the dictionary 'colic' means griping or belly pain (*photo 1*).

There are three common types:

1. *Flatulent colic.* This is the most common and occurs when there is a collection of gas in the bowel. As it passes through, the gas dilates the bowel abnormally and causes a lot of pain. It is the least serious type of colic though it is often the most violent.

2. *Obstructive colic.* This occurs when there is a hard mass of food or faeces in the

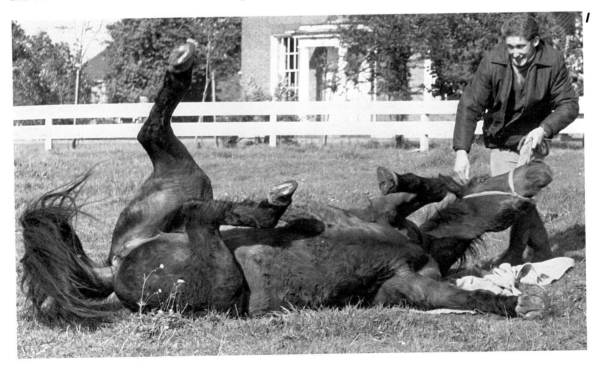

1

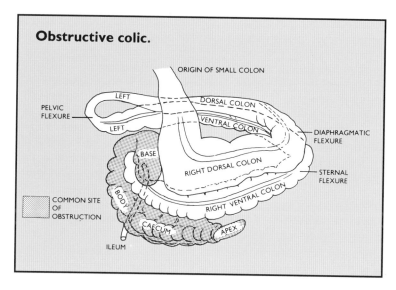

Obstructive colic.

ORIGIN OF SMALL COLON

LEFT

PELVIC FLEXURE

LEFT

DORSAL COLON

VENTRAL COLON

DIAPHRAGMATIC FLEXURE

BASE

RIGHT DORSAL COLON

STERNAL FLEXURE

BODY

RIGHT VENTRAL COLON

COMMON SITE OF OBSTRUCTION

CAECUM

APEX

ILEUM

bowel prohibiting the passage of all materials (*see diagram*).

3. *Twist*. Here the bowel becomes twisted. It is by far the most serious since it is almost invariably fatal.

All these conditions require immediate veterinary attention; the seriousness of the condition cannot be judged by the amount of pain the animal shows.

The best guide is the pulse (*photo 2*); it should beat 35 to 45 times per minute. If it only rises slightly, even though the pain is great, the condition is not serious. If, however, the pulse rises to 80 or 100 it is very serious.

Bright red eye membranes (*photo 3*) are also a characteristic of these conditions.

First-aid precautions

At the first sign of pain all food, including hay, should be removed from the box and the bed made deep and comfortable. A common idea is that the horse should be taken out and kept walking. This is both inadvisable and unkind.

Another common fallacy is that if the horse is allowed to roll, then twist of the bowel will occur. This is not so, horses roll normally and

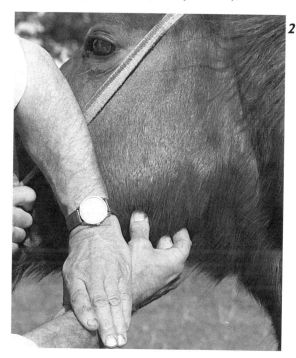

2

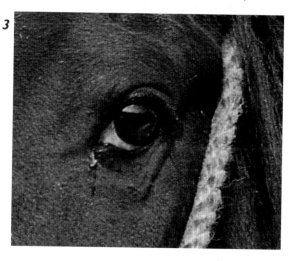

3

healthily and never twist a bowel and they will not do it when they have colic. In a twisted gut the gut is always twisted before the pain starts. Stand by the well-bedded box, and if the horse rolls, all you have to do is to watch he does not get cast and jammed in a corner.

Causes

Most colics result from some form of improper feeding or bad management. Common faults include the following:

1. DIET
Quantity of food. Too little or too much. Ration must be adjusted to work.
Quality of food. Immature or newly-thrashed grain. Damaged foods, e.g. grain overheated in stack; musty hay; dirty food. Poor quality roughage, e.g. chopped straw, oat chaff. Boiled foods and greens such as cabbages may cause tympany.
Irregular feeding. Leads to disordered peristalsis, i.e. bowel movements. Long intervals between meals result in gorging the food without proper mastication.
Sudden changes in diet. For example, immediate introduction to heavy concentrate rations or to young, lush pasture.
Water. Insufficient clean water. Irregular times of watering. Watering when hot, sweating or exhausted.

2. WORK
Excessive work, leading to exhaustion; even moderate work, when not in full training. Irregular work, particularly an idle period followed by a long hard day.
Failure to allow cooling-off period on return.

3. ACCIDENTS
Likely to occur when a horse breaks loose and gorges itself on concentrates.

4. STRONGYLES
Can cause colic especially in thoroughbreds two to four years old (see verminous colic, page 106).

Symptoms

Flatulent colic
This is sometimes called spasmodic colic because the accumulation of gas in the bowel causes pain periodically; there will be quiet spells then violent spells.

The pain in this type of colic is often more extreme than in either of the other two, though the pulse does not rise to more than about 50 (as a rule).

Obstructive colic
The pain is not so severe but is more consistent, often causing the animal to paw (*photo 4*).

The pulse will rise a little higher than in flatulent colic (into the 60s). The impaction can frequently, but not always, be felt by a veterinary surgeon if he examines by rectum.

When he listens to the abdomen with his ear or stethoscope, the lack of normal bowel movements will help him to diagnose this type of colic. Naturally if the bowel is impacted, normal movement is inhibited.

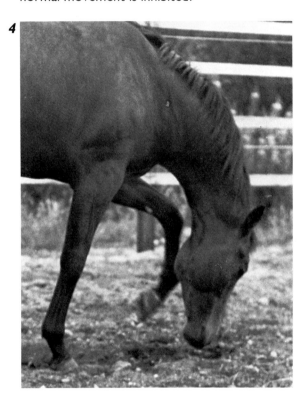

4

Twist colic
The pain to start with is very severe and causes the horse to roll (*photo 5*). It then passes off after a varying length of time, sometimes up to twenty-four hours or even longer, particularly if the twist is in the small bowel as here the area of peritonitis takes that much longer to develop. When the pain passes off, the horse usually breaks into a cold sweat.

The pulse will rise to 120 or thereabouts

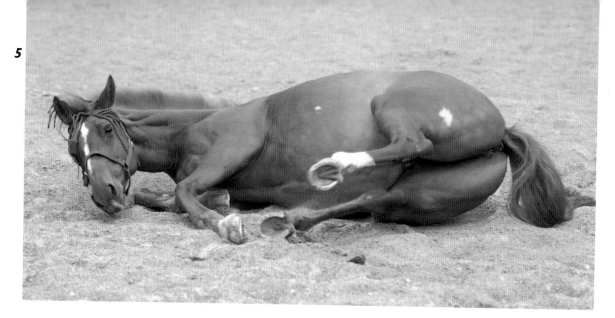

and the animal will just stand and shiver, particularly in the muscles of the shoulder.

There are, of course, other conditions that can cause colic in horses, such as ruptured stomach, peritonitis and kidney troubles, but these are comparatively uncommon and certainly very much a matter for your veterinary surgeon to diagnose and deal with. Grass sickness (see page 108) can of course also cause colic.

Treatment

As mentioned, colic should always be diagnosed and treated by a veterinary surgeon. So-called 'colic drinks' can be purchased but practically all of them contain a sedative which will mask the symptoms and make the veterinary surgeon's diagnosis much more difficult. A twisted gut, caught early, can be cured by operation.

Always confine yourself to the routine first-aid described above. Modern drugs available include antispasmodics and tranquillisers both of which control the pain. These are being continually improved by the drug companies.

Prevention

Study and avoid the causes. Most important is correct feeding and watering. Always remember that the horse's stomach is remarkably small and he must therefore be fed in comparatively small quantities at frequent intervals and, most important of all, at rigidly regular times. Obviously, if the horse is

allowed to go a long time without food or water, he will attack it greedily when he gets it and upset his digestive rhythm. **Fresh water should be available at all times** (photo 6).

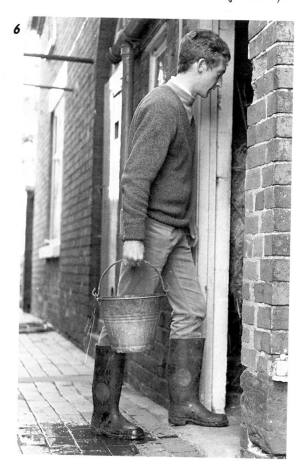

105

Two further observations on colic.

First, a 'dog-like' posture is always a bad sign, that is, when the patient sits up like a dog (*photo 7*). This usually indicates one of the fatal colics due to a ruptured stomach or bowel.

Secondly, renal colic (kidney colic) is not common in the horse, contrary to general opinion. The symptoms are those of abdominal pain, but the pain is nothing like so severe as in the other types of colic. It may be caused by stones or calculi blocking up the ureter or urethra, and there may or may not be blood in the urine. Diagnosis is difficult and should always be left to the veterinary surgeon. He will no doubt examine the urine in a laboratory.

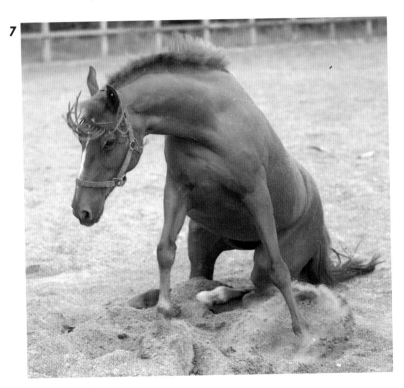

7

52
Verminous Colic

This complaint is found mostly in young horses, especially thoroughbreds two to four years old.

Cause
Massive infestation of roundworms (strongyles) or botts (see pages 45 and 48).

Symptoms
Verminous colic presents a characteristic picture. There occurs persistent or continually recurring colic despite apparently normal bowel sounds.

The patient will eat spasmodically but will drink very little water.

He will repeatedly paw the air with one or other foreleg (*photo 1*) and gaze round pathetically at his flank (*photo 2*).

The pulse and eye may remain fairly good, but the horse rapidly loses condition and the pain will persist for days or even weeks if the condition is not correctly diagnosed and treated promptly.

Treatment

A veterinary surgeon is needed to diagnose and treat such cases. He will probably use the stomach pump against the botts and prescribe a powerful anthelmintic to destroy the roundworms. Symptoms of indigestion may persist for several days after the dosing, but the bouts of pain should become progressively less frequent and less severe.

Prevention

Never forget to dose for worms every six weeks. The young horses require particular

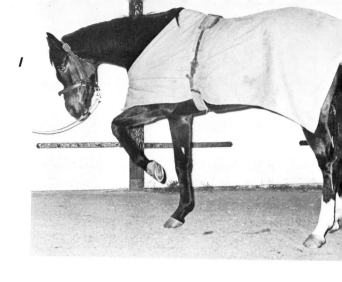

attention.

For the winter dosing it is a good idea to choose an anthelmintic that will act against botts as well as against roundworms. Dichlorvos does this double job extremely well, as do several other easily given proprietary preparations.

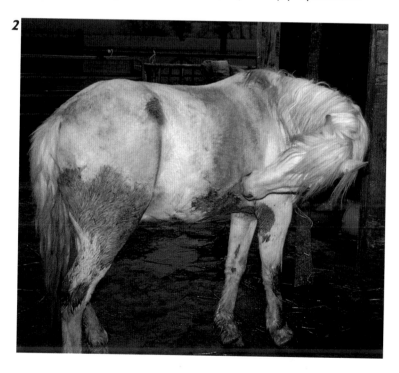

53
Grass Sickness

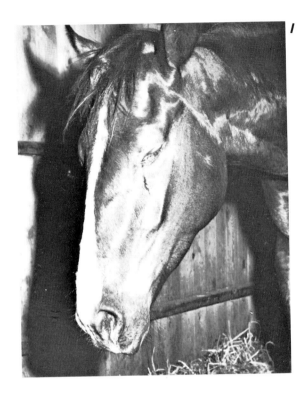

occasional cases occur but these can and do appear throughout the entire country.

Symptoms
The case may be either acute or sub-acute.

Acute grass sickness
When the acute disease strikes, the condition is easily mistaken for colic since the first symptoms are those of acute abdominal pain with the other signs that go with it, namely, sweating (this may be patchy), muscle tremors (shivering), accelerated pulse and respirations (*photo 2*).

A complete stasis or stoppage of the bowel occurs. This is due to paralysis of the bowel wall; in fact, the paralysis is so complete that no movement can be heard by listening at the flanks.

Death will occur in 48 to 72 hours with the pulse very similar to that in a fatal colic, e.g. twisted gut.

Grass sickness is probably the most deadly of all horse conditions (*photo 1*).

Cause
The precise cause is still unknown, but it is the opinion of many of the modern scientists that grass sickness will eventually prove to be due to a virus infection.

In the early 1920s grass sickness became practically epidemic on the east coast of Scotland. At that time farm horses were in common use and the entire horse population was almost wiped out. Since then, fortunately, the disease has become endemic, i.e. ever-present but quiescent. This means that only

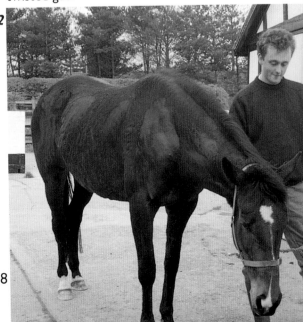

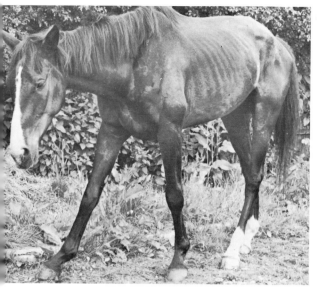

Sub-acute grass sickness
In a sub-acute case (*photo 3*), the patient may linger on for three or four weeks or even longer. Just occasionally the odd horse might eventually recover, but if it does, it is usually a

3 hopeless wreck.

In the sub-acute form the initial bowe is followed by a spreading of the paralysi throughout the entire alimentary tract. T animal becomes unable to swallow; if it attempts to drink or suck in some water, the water runs back down through the nostrils. The breath smells vile.

As the case advances and there is still no passage through the bowel irrespective of what medicines are given, a froth or soapiness appears under the dock and around the tail. This is practically diagnostic.

The animal becomes more and more 'tucked up' ('herring-gutted'), and this 'tucking-up' continues to get worse until death supervenes.

Treatment
No satisfactory treatment has been discovered and it is my opinion that, until such times as the precise cause is discovered, it is much better to resort to humane slaughter as soon as the disease is diagnosed.

54
Rabies

I am often asked if horses can get rabies. The answer is yes if they are bitten by a rabid dog, fox, monkey etc.

Symptoms
Approximately six weeks after the bite the horse develops a colic which fails to respond to painkillers or muscle-relaxants. This is followed by attacks of violent excitement with kicking and head throwing but no sweating.

After three or four days the head swells, the patient has difficulty in standing and refuses to drink.

Brain symptoms — unco-ordinated movements etc. — develop shortly before death.

Fortunately, affected horses rarely become aggressive, so they are not liable to spread the disease.

55
Enteritis

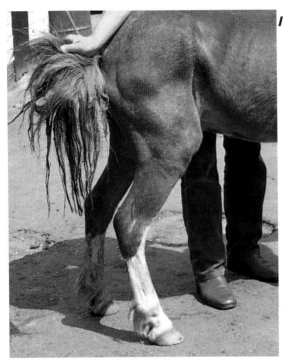

Enteritis simply means inflammation of the bowel or intestinal lining. When this happens the peristaltic waves that are continually passing along the intestinal wall become accelerated and force the bowel contents along much faster than normal. The glands in the wall of the intestine secrete an excess of fluid; at the same time the intestinal wall does not absorb the usual quantity of fluid because it doesn't get the time or the chance. The result produces the typical signs of enteritis.

Symptoms
In the acute stages, spasmodic pain and diarrhoea; this may be copious, so much so that the horse may appear to pass nothing more or less than hot water (*photo 1*).

Causes
These are varied. They may be:
Bacterial
Dietetic — e.g. the animal may have eaten mouldy hay, bran, or oats — all of which may contain fungi that can cause a very acute enteritis (*photo 2*).
Chemical — e.g. lead from chewing paint.
Vegetable — e.g. certain poisonous plants which may be eaten during grazing.

Treatment
Enteritis can be one of the most serious of all equine complaints, so send for your veterinary surgeon at once. Never try 'do-it-yourself' treatments on a horse with diarrhoea.

If at grass, bring the patient up into a warm box, rug him up and leave the diagnosis and treatment to your veterinary surgeon. His first concern will be to try to establish the cause. Having done so, he will prescribe

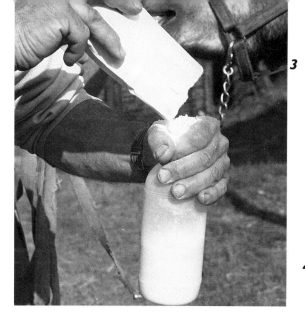

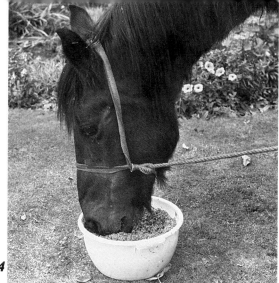

antispasmodics, sedatives and probably antibiotics.

Never give purgatives. They may produce a fatal superpurgation or dysentery. If the veterinary surgeon is not immediately available, kaolin in fairly large quantities shaken up in water is always safe and does form a protective covering over the inflamed bowel surface (*photo 3*), and the water the horse gets with the kaolin helps to replace some of the fluid lost in the diarrhoea. Like all animals, the horse is susceptible to dehydration (i.e. loss of body fluids) which can in itself cause

death. It may well be necessary for your veterinary surgeon to inject fluid intravenously in the form of normal saline solution or glucose. Chloradyne (tincture of chloroform and morphine) or one of the other old-fashioned astringents may be beneficial after the acute stages.

After-treatment
The recovering and convalescent patient should be introduced very gradually to its food. Bran mashes are undoubtedly the best to begin with — three times a day for at least three days (*photo 4*).

56
Colitis

Colitis means inflammation of the colon or main part of the large intestine.

Cause
Seen mainly in young animals during or after a heavy infestation of roundworm (*photo 1*). In certain cases a severe or chronic colitis follows dosing with certain worm remedies, resulting in the development of a chronic diarrhoea.

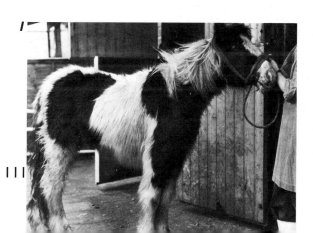

Treatment
Extremely difficult and should be left entirely to a veterinary surgeon. Stomach pumping with 2 kg of sieved normal horse's faeces may be the only cure.

Prevention
Regular dosing against roundworms. Young foals at pasture should be dosed every six weeks from the age of two months throughout the rest of their lives.

57
Salmonellosis

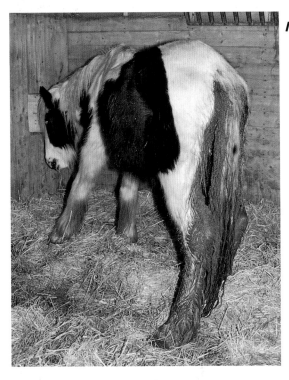

Cause
Several species of the salmonella organism but especially the *Salmonella typhimurium*.

Predisposing causes
Lowered resistance by disease, malnutrition, or in the case of foals by deficiency of colostral intake or having dirty navels.

Heavy worm infestation.

Stress due to long journeys or surgical operations.

Build-up of infection in dirty loose boxes.

Symptoms
In young foals generalised septicaemia and death. In older foals from one to three months a suppurative joint-ill or a diarrhoea which fails to respond to routine antibiotic treatment.

In colts, fillies and older horses persistent scouring (*photo 1*), rapid loss in condition, dehydration and often septicaemia, all of which symptoms often get progressively worse despite treatment.

Treatment
A veterinary surgeon will of course have to confirm the diagnosis and type the bacterium. Treatment is by antibiotics and sulpha drugs given both orally and by injection, but is mostly unsuccessful, although mild cases may recover.

Prevention
Make certain foals get their full quota of colostrum and dress the navel carefully against infection. From two months onwards dose every six weeks for worms. Feed carefully and well especially during the winter. Scrub out loose boxes regularly with hot water and washing soda.

Note
Salmonella presents a public health hazard and all positive cases must be reported to the Ministry of Agriculture.

58
Nephritis (Inflammation of the Kidneys)

Kidney inflammation (called nephritis) is comparatively uncommon in the young horse, but it is my experience that chronic nephritis often occurs in horses and ponies from the age of fifteen or sixteen years onwards. The condition is more common in mares than in geldings, especially if they have been used for breeding. The patient illustrated was just over 20 years old (*photo 1*).

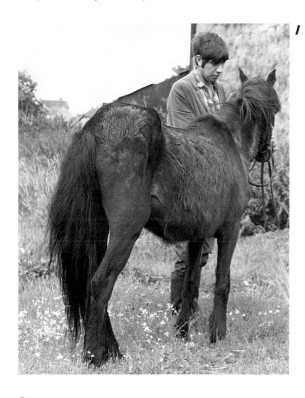

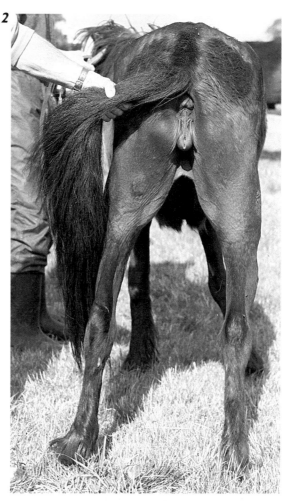

Symptoms
Progressive loss in condition despite a good appetite (*photo 2*). Many owners repeatedly treat such cases for worms with, of course, no success whatsoever.

The reason why the affected pony becomes emaciated is because the protein (that should be used to repair and build up muscles and tissues) is excreted through the damaged kidneys into the urine instead of being passed to the liver for the body's utilisation.

After a few weeks well-marked ulcers often

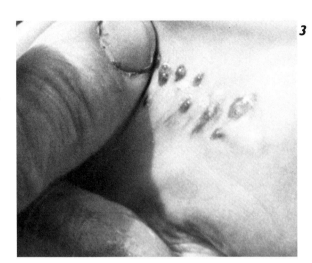

appear in the pony's mouth (*photo 3*).

Treatment
Send for your veterinary surgeon. He will take blood and urine samples, assess the amount of damage and prescribe treatment if at all possible.

It is my experience that chronic nephritis cases rarely respond to treatment; sooner or later the patient goes down and is unable to rise. Painless euthanasia is then indicated.

MALNUTRITION

One condition that may be mistaken for chronic nephritis is malnutrition, and this should always be suspected if the horse or pony is comparatively young (*photo 4*).

Symptoms
The same progressive loss in condition with almost invariably well-marked ulcers in the mouth. In fact such ulcers are a diagnostic feature of starvation, as also is acute anemia (*photo 5*).

Treatment and prevention
Follow carefully the feeding instructions given in Chapter 17 and dose the outlying horses and ponies for worms every six weeks — winter and summer.

At the same time dust the malnourished animal with a reputable parasitic powder once a week for three or four weeks since horse lice thrive on such animals.

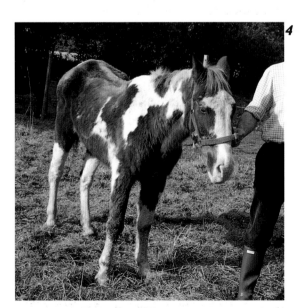

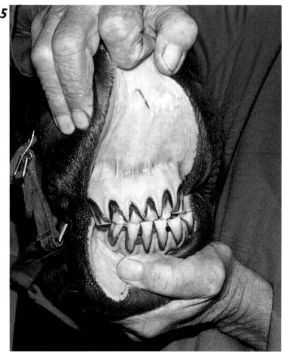

Legs

59
Lameness

Lameness is generally an indication of pain in one or more legs. There is, however, one other type of lameness, i.e. a mechanical lameness. This arises when there is a stiffness of a joint or a contraction of a tendon whereby, mechanically, the horse is unable to move his leg in a normal manner and is definitely lame though suffering no pain.

In normal lameness due to pain, the first thing to find out is which is the lame leg. To do this, have the horse walked away from you, then back towards you; then have him trotted away and back. Do not look at the horse's legs in the first instance, watch his head, especially as he comes towards you; keep your eyes fixed on the poll between the ears (*photo 1*).

If the head 'nods', then this confirms the horse is lame. Now widen your field of vision to take in the forelegs — the horse will **nod onto the sound leg**. This is simply because he is getting onto the sound leg quicker than normal — taking a short step with his lame leg and nodding quickly onto the sound leg.

If both forelegs move freely, fix your eyes on the **quarters** as the horse moves away from you (*photo 2*). If the lameness is behind, then one quarter drops more than the other. That again is the **sound** leg on which he is dropping. The lame leg is the higher quarter.

If you have decided that the horse is lame in front and which leg he is lame on, then have him trotted towards you again, this time

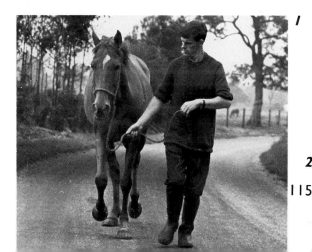

1

2

115

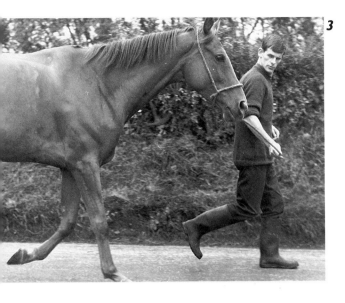

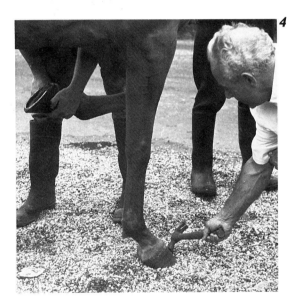

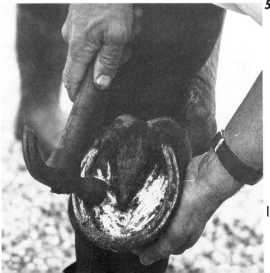

3 watching the legs only. If the lame leg moves straight forward in a normal way but with a shorter step than the sound leg, then the chances are he is lame low down.

If, on the other hand, he swings the leg outwards, not bending it properly, then the chances are he is lame higher up, probably in the shoulder.

Now stand to the side and watch the horse trot past you; keep an eagle eye on the solar surface of his foot to see if he is landing square or on his toe or heel (*photo 3*). If he is landing on his heel, the lameness is most likely to be in front; if on his toe, the back of the leg is probably involved.

Examining the individual leg for lameness

4 *Always start at the foot and always examine the foot, no matter where you think the lameness may be.* Have the sound leg lifted and tap the suspect foot all around with a hammer (*photo 4*).

Then let the other forefoot down; lift the affected one and tap all round the sole (*photo 5*). **If the patient evinces any pain,** call your veterinary surgeon immediately. He will have the shoe removed (*photo 6*), and will search the foot carefully for a picked-up nail, a puncture, or an abscess.

If there is no sign of pain in the foot, start at the hoof head and work gradually up looking for any sign of swelling, pain, or abnormality.

The fetlock joint should be put into complete flexion and held that way for some time (*photo 7*), then the horse should be trotted on. If the lameness is more marked, the joint surface is probably involved. If no **5** result, repeat in turn with the knee, the elbow and the shoulder.

With a hind-leg lameness, follow the exact procedure (*photo 8*). Unfortunately, however, it is impossible to bend the hock without bending the stifle, and this makes it extremely difficult to differentiate between a hock and a stifle lameness.

Obviously, the diagnosis of lameness requires a great deal of skill and experience, and is indeed a job that should be left to the veterinary surgeon. Nonetheless, by following the simple rules I have given, it is possible to

116

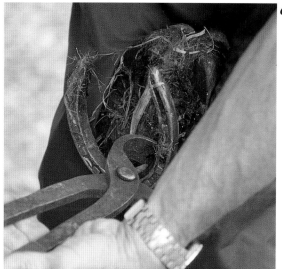

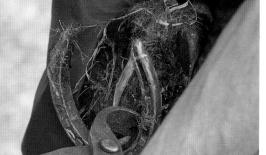

6 make an intelligent guess. All amateurs love to test their knowledge and it provides a great deal of pleasure to have an 'intelligent guess' subsequently confirmed by the professional.

8

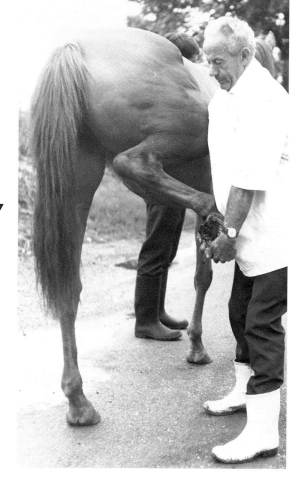

7

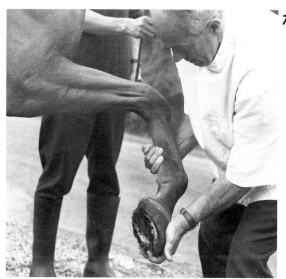

60
Shoulder Lameness

It has been my experience over the years that most so-called shoulder lamenesses eventually turn out to be due to navicular disease (see page 162). However, shoulder lameness can and does occur (*photo 1*).

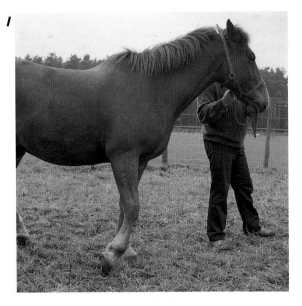

Cause
Usually direct injury which produces a painful swelling round the joint; causes an inflammation of the bursa situated between the tendon of the biceps and the humerus; or damages the suprascapular or radial nerve.

Symptoms
Apart from any obvious swelling or pain, typical signs include:
1. A sharp raising of the head when the patient tries to bring the leg forward at the walk or trot.
2. A short stride with the affected leg held almost straight, causing in many cases stumbling.
3. Fixation of the shoulder (scapulohumeral) joint when the horse tries to move. In other words it tends to swing the leg outward and forward with only partial flexion (*photo 2*).
4. Dropped elbow if the radial nerve is damaged (see next chapter) or wasting of the muscles when the suprascapular nerve is damaged.

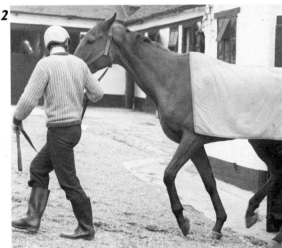

Treatment
Initially cortisone injections help to ease the pain and reduce the swelling, but the best treatment of all is prolonged rest.

Recently swimming therapy has apparently given beneficial results; certainly, general physiotherapy after a period of rest does help considerably.

61
Radial Paralysis

The patient suffers partial or complete paralysis of the radial nerve which passes over the front of the shoulder before descending into the foreleg.

Cause

Usually direct injury to the front of the horse's shoulder.

Symptoms

The elbow is dropped and the front toe is dragged (*photo 1*). There are usually ample signs of trauma or swelling around the shoulder joint.

After the swelling subsides, the dropped elbow and toe dragging may persist for three to six months or even longer depending on the amount of damage to the nerve.

Treatment

Complete rest and cortisone injections until all the swelling and pain have subsided.

Thereafter, if in the summer, turn the patient out to graze and exercise the utmost patience.

Modern physiotherapy can help such conditions tremendously, so it is always best to consult your veterinary surgeon.

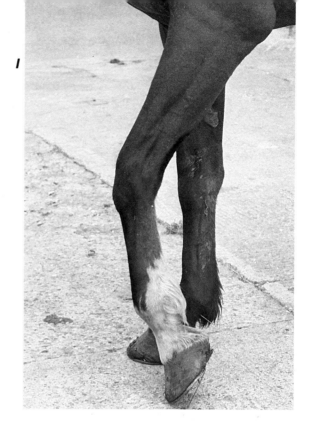

62
Spavin

A spavin is a hard bony swelling (similar to a ringbone) or callosity which occurs on the antero-internal aspect of the hock, that is, at the front, inside, and lower edge of the hock joint (*photo 1*). It involves the lower bone of the tarsus and the head of the metatarsus.

Symptoms

The hard bony swelling is usually accompanied by a chronic or recurrent lameness. This lameness is accentuated when the hock is flexed tightly (*photo 2*).

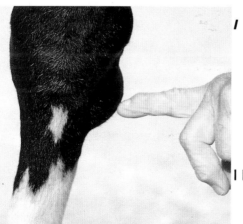

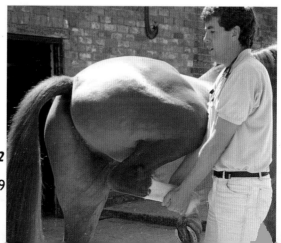

Causes

Strain or sprain, or direct trauma or injury, either of which can cause an inflammation on the surface of the bone which leads to a new growth of bone — an exostosis. Often the damage encroaches on the joint surface producing an arthritis.

Treatment

1. Complete rest; as in all inflammations and sprains, rest is far and away the most important factor in healng.

2. The operation of cunean tendonectomy comprising the removal of 1-1½ inches of the cunean tendon which passes over the spavin area. Excision of the tendon removes one source of pain and in some cases produces soundness (*photo 3*). I have had successes with this treatment.

3. There is little or nothing to be gained by blistering or by repeated applications of iodine preparations or embrocation.

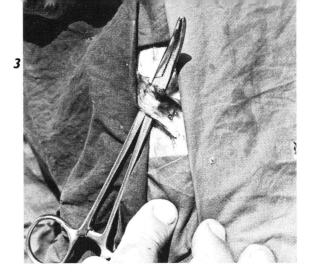

4. Deep point firing after varying periods of rest. The main object in firing is to enforce rest but it also assists in the full formation of the callosity or exostosis. I don't like this treatment and would recommend it only as a last resort. The practice is now frowned upon by the British veterinary profession.

63
Gonitis

Gonitis simply means inflammation of the stifle joint. It is probably the worst of all the horse lamenesses simply because the stifle joint, which is the equivalent of the human knee joint, is very complicated in structure (*see diagram*).

Cause

Direct injury, sprained, torn or ruptured ligaments, injuries to the cartilages or menisci, trauma (bruising) or puncture of the joint capsule.

Symptoms

The outstanding symptom of gonitis is that the horse goes on the toe of the injured leg (*photo 1*). He also rests the leg with the toe

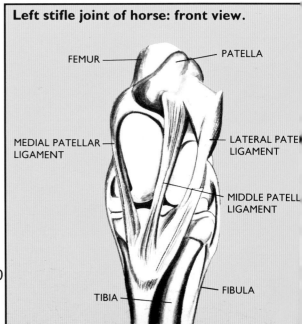

Left stifle joint of horse: front view.

FEMUR — — PATELLA

MEDIAL PATELLAR LIGAMENT

LATERAL PATE[LLAR] LIGAMENT

MIDDLE PATELL[AR] LIGAMENT

TIBIA — — FIBULA

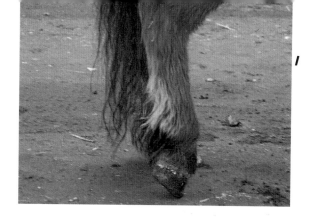

on the ground and the fetlock joint pushed forward in an attempt to alleviate pressure on his stifle. The affected stifle joint is usually swollen and painful and the pain is intensified when the joint is flexed.

Treatment
Prolonged rest is the only hope. The prognosis is bad. The end result is usually chronic lameness.

64
Luxated Patella

Perhaps the most common predisposing cause of gonitis is a luxated or luxating patella (*photo 1*). The patella is the knee cap, and luxation simply means displacement. Usually in the horse the luxating patella moves in and out of position either inwards (medial luxation) or outwards (lateral luxation) according to which ligament is damaged. Occasionally it locks in an upward position.

Cause
The patella is held in position by three powerful ligaments (*see diagram on facing page*). Luxation occurs when one or other of the outside ligaments become torn or damaged. This is most likely to occur when the horse is in poor condition.

Symptoms
When moving forward the patient drags his toe forward (*photo 2*), and the patella clicks

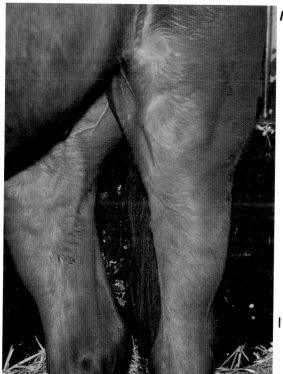

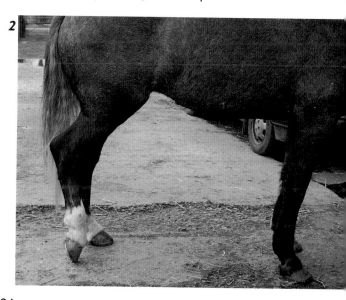

back into position when he takes full weight on the leg. Occasionally the moving patella can be heard, but usually it is seen by watching the stifle joint closely when the horse walks on.

Treatment
Complete rest is the most valuable of all treatments, but the rest period has to be prolonged for up to one year or even longer. At the same time the patient's general condition must be improved by regular and correct feeding.

If the horse is valuable, it is worthwhile trying orthopaedic surgery, but the case must be placed in the hands of the surgeon at the earliest possible moment so that the overall joint damage will be minimal.

The operation comprises section and fixation of the appropriate ligament. I have performed it on several occasions, but my success rate has been moderate probably because of the weight of the patients.

Prognosis
With all cases of luxation the prognosis is not good. It has always been my experience that most damaged stifle joints remain a source of potential trouble.

For this reason, if the patient is a mare or a stallion it is best to retire it to stud.

65
Ringbone

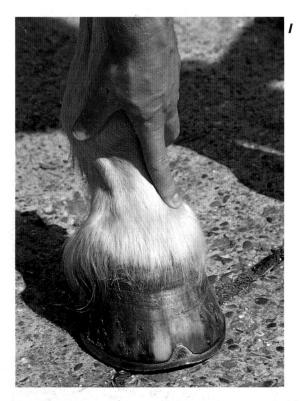

A ringbone is an exostosis — that is a growth of new bone on the surface of an original bone (*photo 1*).

It occurs on the pastern and it may be a 'high' ringbone or a 'low' ringbone.

In high ringbone the first phalanx is involved — that is the bone that runs from the fetlock to the first joint below the fetlock (*photo 2*).

In low ringbone the second phalanx is involved — just above or, in very serious cases, below the top of the hoof (*photo 3*).

There are also 'articular' and 'non-articular' ringbones.

By 'articular' is simply meant that the ringbone involves the joint either between the 1st and 2nd phalanx or between the 2nd and 3rd phalanx (the 3rd phalanx is the bone of the hoof — the pedal bone); that is, the joint at the top of the hoof (*photo 4*).

When it occurs
Ringbone may occur at any age — it is seen in young horses, yearlings, and can appear in old horses.

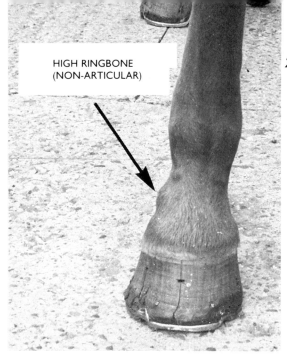

HIGH RINGBONE
(NON-ARTICULAR)

2 Causes

Trauma — direct injury.
Concussion — constant banging on hard roads.
Hereditary predisposition (undoubtedly exists).
Defects in conformation causing bad shoeing.
Improper foot balance.

Symptoms

Marked lameness. Diagnosis is made on the lameness plus the appearance of a painful swelling over the affected area.

After varying periods of time of up to several months, the pain on palpation will disappear and a callous or new bone formation will form.

In non-articular lameness, when the callosity or bone is completely formed, the lameness will go and the chances are that it will not return.

3 In articular ringbone, however, the prognosis is very grave and lameness may be permanent because the roughness of the callous formation may, and very often does, extend onto the joint itself.

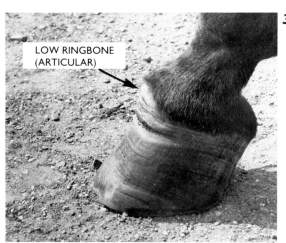

LOW RINGBONE
(ARTICULAR)

Treatment

In the first instance, complete rest for periods of up to an entire season.

Later, if lameness still persists, deep point firing and blistering may be tried (*photo 5*); though in articular ringbone there is very little chance of complete success.

Nothing is to be gained by the repeated rubbing of the swelling with iodine preparations or embrocation.

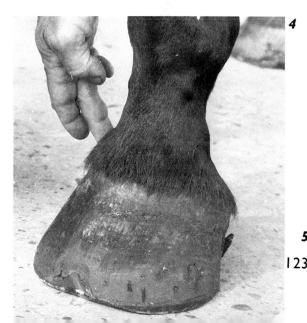

4

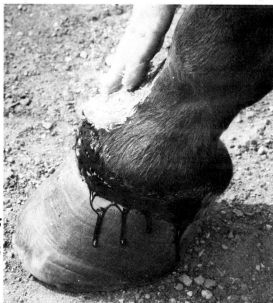

5

66
Itchy Heels

This is seen chiefly in the autumn.

Cause
Larvae of the harvest mite. These larvae come off the grasses or herbage, and though they live only for a few days in the horse's heels, they can and do cause considerable irritation. Sometimes the mite spreads its activities to around the coronary band (*photo 1*).

Symptoms
Foot stamping (*photo 2*) and nibbling.

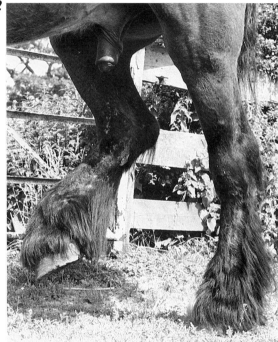

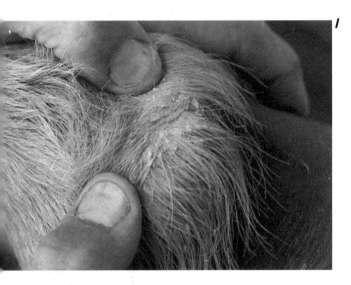

Treatment and prevention
Dress the lower parts of the horse's legs once a week from the first of September to the middle of November with an anti-parasitic dusting powder or a gammexane bath, which is probably more effective, especially if it is scrubbed in with a hard bristle brush.

67
Splints

In order to understand exactly what splints are, some knowledge of simple anatomy is essential.

Consider the metacarpus or cannon bone which runs from the knee to the fetlock.

At the back of the cannon bone and to each side of it lie the two small metacarpal bones or 'splint bones'. They are broad at the top, where they form part of the knee joint, and taper to a point about two thirds of the way down the cannon bone (*see diagram A*).

Each of these two 'splint bones' is attached to the periosteum, or covering of the cannon bone, by a ligament. When there is any excess stress or strain on the forelegs, one or other of the ligaments may become stretched or sprained and when this happens the periosteum is pulled away from the bone.

The resultant inflammation causes swelling, local pain and often marked lameness. The pain and lameness will pass off in two or three weeks, but the swelling will become harder simply because the inflammatory fluid and tissue change into bone. In doing so, it unites the splint bone directly to the cannon bone.

Commonest position
The commonest position for splints is to the outside of the upper third of the cannon and splint bone (*photo 1*).

Diagram A
Rear view of cannon bone.

SMALL
METACARPAL OR
SPLINT BONE

METACARPUS OR
CANNON BONE

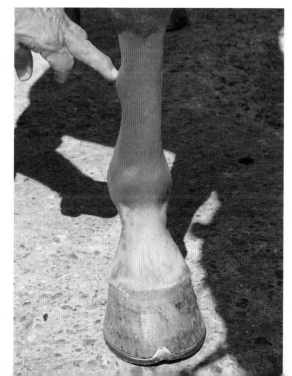

1

More serious positions

The splint may form on the inside of the splint bone (*photo 2*) and it can then be serious because its presence, even after it has settled down, can interfere with the action of the suspensory and check ligaments which run down the back of the cannon bone between the two splint bones.

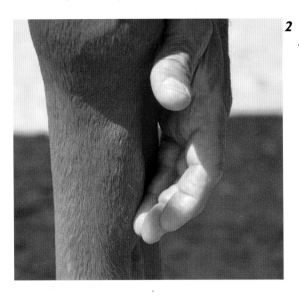

2

When an extensive splint forms across the back of the cannon bone underneath the flexor tendons, it is sometimes called a *rod splint* (*see diagram B*). When the splint forms

**Diagram B
A rod splint.**

SPLINT EXTENDING UNDER THE FLEXOR TENDONS

at the head of the splint bone, it can become a very serious condition because it can involve, and interfere with the action of, the knee joint. This is called a *jack splint*.

When they occur

Splints most frequently appear in young horses (three to four years old) when they start serious work (*photo 3*).

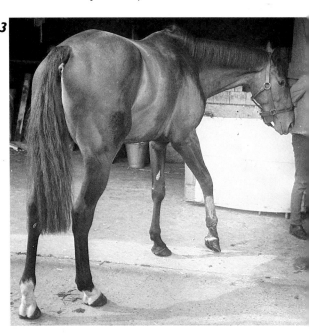

3

Symptoms

Lameness. Swelling and pain on pressure over the seat or spot where the splint is developing.

Treatment

Rest is essential until the lameness is gone. This can take up to three or even four weeks.

During the first week of the rest period, kaolin poultices should be applied to the part twice daily (*photo 4*).

A slightly more spectacular treatment comprises injections of cortisone into the swelling, while many pin their faith on blistering, or point firing and blistering.

It is my opinion that the poulticing and rest are adequate. They are certainly logical and sensible because time, and time alone, heals satisfactorily. One has to wait until the bone callosity is completely formed.

After the lameness disappears, work must

126

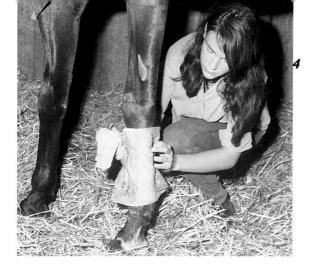

4 be introduced only very gradually; otherwise the ligament may tear again and set back the convalescence another month.

Are splints an unsoundness?
The average splint is not a serious condition but it can, and does, spoil the look of a show animal, and some judges will downgrade the affected horse or pony immediately.

Technically speaking, however, a splint does not comprise an unsoundness unless it is on the line of the tendons or interfering with the action of the joint.

68
Arthritis

True arthritis is comparatively uncommon in the horse but when it occurs it usually affects the majority if not all of the joints in the body (*photo 1*).

Symptoms
The horse comes out of the box markedly lame especially in cold weather. Often it is difficult or impossible to tell which leg is

1

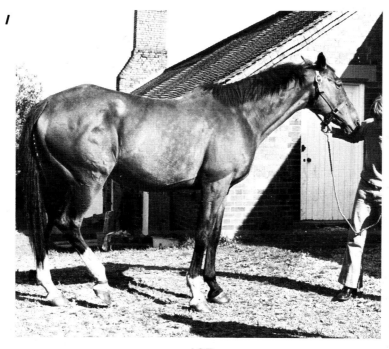

affected since two, three or all four legs may be stiff.

The condition improves with exercise but some lameness persists permanently.

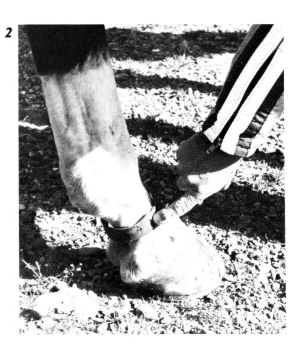

Diagnosis
This can only be confirmed by X-ray.

Prognosis
Very bad. The condition becomes progressively worse despite any form of therapy.

Treatment
In the early stages, a prolonged course of phenylbutazone may make the animal workable for a time but the relief is only transient.

Quack treatments such as copper bands interwoven in leather anklets (*photo 2*) are of psychological value only.

69
Sprained Flexor Tendons

Running down the back of the cannon bones are the two flexor tendons — the superficial and the deep (*see diagram*). Their function is to bend the legs when the muscles at their upper end contract.

When the horse is galloping or jumping and extending his legs forward to the complete extremity, each time his forefeet land the strain on the flexor tendons (and on the suspensory ligament — see Sprain of the Suspensory Ligament, page 138) is immense (*photo 1*). Frequently, some of the fibres of the tendon give way or, in an extreme case, the whole tendon may rupture.

A chronic sprain can lead to a bowed tendon (*photo 2*).

Symptoms
In the average case, where only part of one tendon is involved, the usual symptoms are marked lameness, swelling and puffiness over the affected part and distinct pain on palpation (*photo 3*).

Treatment
Complete rest for a long period, usually at least for the remainder of the season and certainly for a minimum of three months.

In the early stages, twice-daily kaolin poulticing and bandaging is advisable until the pain and swelling have subsided (*photo 4*).

If the swelling is excessive, the fluid contents can be aspirated by your veterinary surgeon

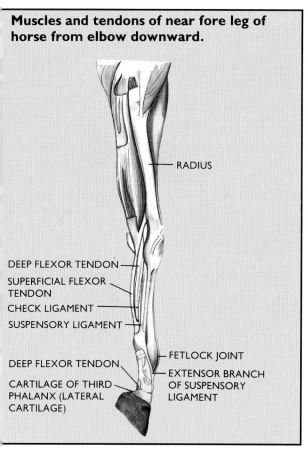

Muscles and tendons of near fore leg of horse from elbow downward.

RADIUS

DEEP FLEXOR TENDON

SUPERFICIAL FLEXOR TENDON

CHECK LIGAMENT

SUSPENSORY LIGAMENT

FETLOCK JOINT

DEEP FLEXOR TENDON

EXTENSOR BRANCH OF SUSPENSORY LIGAMENT

CARTILAGE OF THIRD PHALANX (LATERAL CARTILAGE)

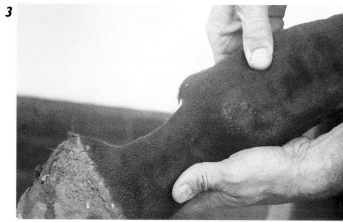

2

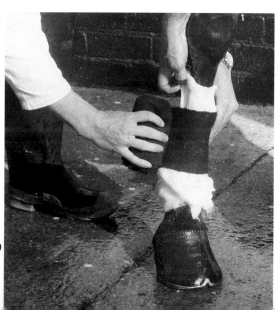

3

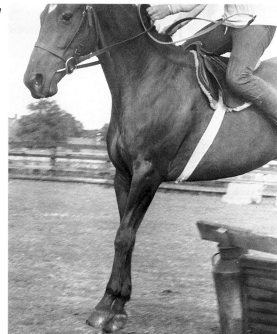

1

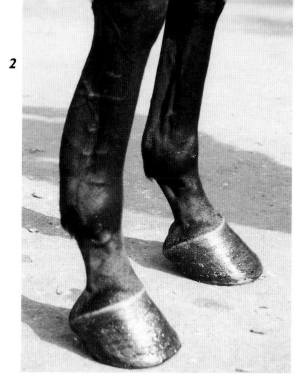

4

who will probably inject special cortisone into the area after the aspiration (*photo 5*).

If the tendons are completely ruptured, then the fetlock will be on the ground. Such cases are hopeless.

After the pain has completely subsided, deep point firing may be resorted to (*photo 6*). This rather drastic treatment, for some reason or other, seems to be successful in many cases despite the fact that many veterinary surgeons are opposed to it. It may be that the success of the treatment is due mainly to the enforced prolonged rest.

There are numerous methods of firing — line, point or acid-firing — and the efficacy of each method is debatable. Certainly the tendon or ligament that has once been strained is never as good again and is always liable to break down with work.

It is to be hoped that, in the future, the development of tendon section operations and equine physiotherapy will obviate the necessity for firing. As stated earlier, the practice of firing is now being outlawed by the British veterinary profession. Personally I feel firing is justified when the only alternative is euthanasia.

One other very valuable treatment now widely used is swimming (*photo 7*).

5

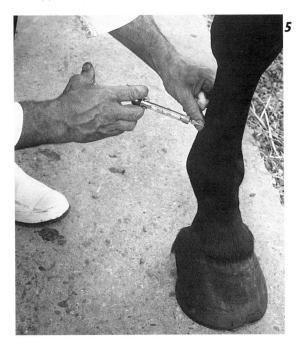

6

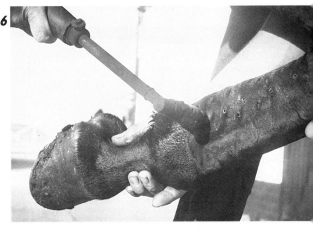

7

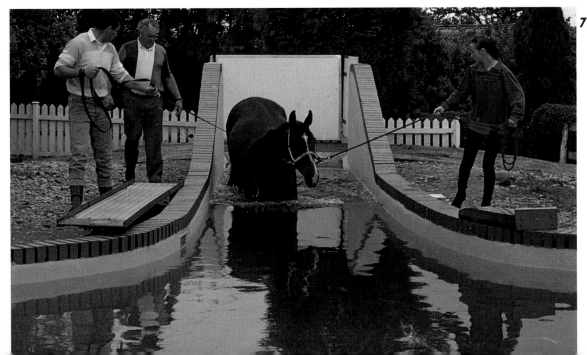

70
Slipped Flexor Tendons

The superficial flexor tendons of the hind legs pass over the point of the hocks and are held in position by lateral ligaments. If or when any of these lateral ligaments are torn by injury or by excess work on heavy ground, then the flexor tendon may slip to the outside of the hock, producing the condition of slipped flexor tendon (*photo 1*).

Symptoms
An initial lameness which may last for several weeks. The displaced tendon can easily be identified.

Treatment
Complete rest. When the pain has gone the tendon adjusts itself to its new position and the horse can resume work without lameness, being gradually brought back to galloping and jumping.

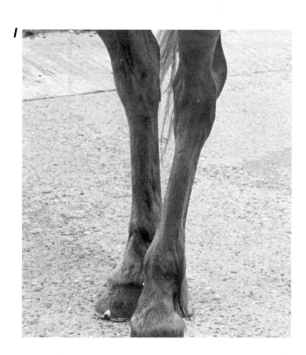

71
Synovial Distensions

Synovia is a fluid that is discharged by synovial membranes, which line the inside of the joints. In addition, they line the sheaths which fit around the tendons and also numerous small pockets or sacs in various parts of the body — sacs that are called 'bursae'.

The synovia acts as a lubricant to keep the joints working smoothly, to keep the tendons moving smoothly in their sheaths and to lubricate the bursae so that they may satisfactorily glide either over a point of bone or round a corner.

If, for any reason, the synovial membrane becomes inflamed in part or in whole, then it

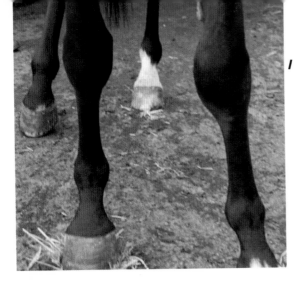

I will discharge more than the normal quantity of fluid into the joint, tendon sheath or bursa and a swelling — usually non-painful — will result. Such a swelling is known as a synovial distension (*photo 1*). When a bursa is involved, the condition is described as a bursitis.

Bog spavin

This is a synovial swelling that appears on the inside of the hock towards the front, but higher than the site of ordinary spavin (*photo 2*). The swelling is soft and non-painful.

Does it comprise an unsoundness?
Yes.

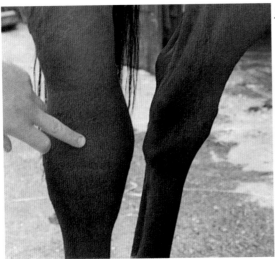

2

Is there any satisfactory treatment?
If no lameness is present, it is best to leave well alone.

It is wise to have the joint X-rayed to make sure there is no bone damage (*photo 3*).

Boggy hock

This occurs when the whole joint capsule is involved and the swelling is uniform around the hock (*photo 4*). It is non-painful.

Boggy hock frequently occurs in young horses at grass and can be associated with an invasion of the leg arteries by strongyle larvae. Usually, however, when the young animals are brought up and put to work the swelling disappears.

3 In old horses, unfortunately, the swelling does not disappear and in most cases it becomes permanent.

A boggy hock is definitely an unsoundness, even though it is not usually associated with lameness.

Treatment
If not lame, leave well alone; if lame, send for your veterinary surgeon. If a young horse, dose for worms.

Capped hock

At the point of the hock there is a bursa; this occasionally becomes enlarged and filled with fluid. When it does it is known as a capped hock (*photo 5*).

When the bursa in front of the knee is affected, a capped knee is the result (*photo 6*).

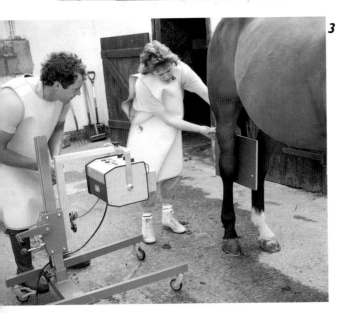

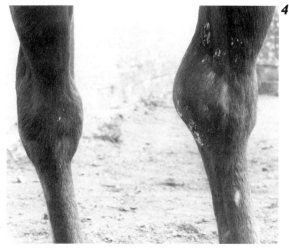

4 Cause

An injury — produced perhaps by the horse kicking at a stable wall or at any hard object; or perhaps by repeated knocking on a hard or slippery stable or loose box floor in attempts to get up.

In the early stages, since it is the result of an injury, it is painful because of the general bruising, but the fluid in the bursa does not give rise to pain though it usually persists and leaves some permanent swelling.

However, capped hock is not an unsoundness, though it must be mentioned on a veterinary certificate.

Treatment

5 When it first happens, the cold hose twice daily is as good a treatment as any, but after the pain has subsided it is futile to apply any treatment, especially since capped hock is not an unsoundness — only a blemish.

Thoroughpin

Just above the hock, both on the inside and on the outside and to the back of the hock, run two tendon sheaths. These frequently become distended with synovial fluid and the resultant swelling is known as a thoroughpin (*photo 7*).

Like capped hock, a thoroughpin is not an unsoundness, only a blemish, and, again, the best treatment is to leave well alone.

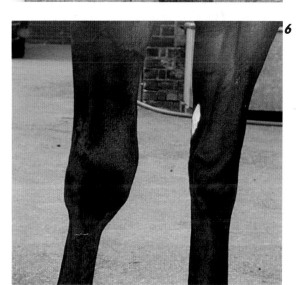

6

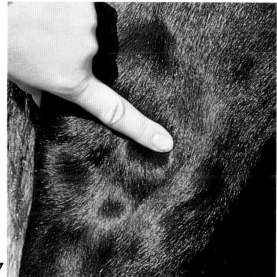

7

Windgalls

Above the fetlocks on the inside and on the outside are two tendon sheaths. When these become filled and dilated with synovial fluid, they produce the condition known as windgalls (*photo 8*).

Windgalls occur most frequently in older horses and can affect both the fore and the hind legs. They may be an unsightly blemish but they are not classified as an unsoundness.

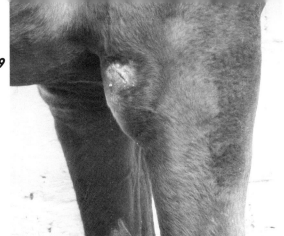

9

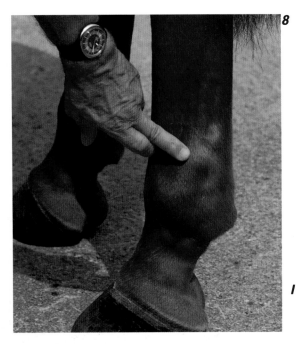

8

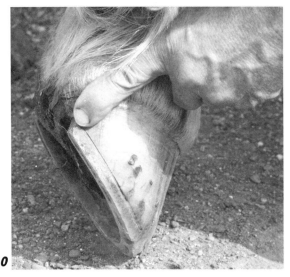

10

Capped elbow

On the point of the elbow there is another bursa. Certain horses or ponies, when getting up or down, strike the point of the elbow with the heel of their fore shoe. This produces a synovial swelling within the bursa and gives rise to the condition called a capped elbow or an elbow gall (*photo 9*).

The way to prevent capped elbow is to keep the feet regularly shod with the heels not too long (*photo 10*).

General treatment of synovial distensions

Treatment of any or all of the synovial distensions is not of much avail, except in the early inflammatory stages (see 'Capped hock').

The distensions can be aspirated (the fluid drawn off with a needle) and injected with various preparations, the most popular being intra-articular cortisone.

However, since the capsule of the distension still remains, nature will rapidly fill it up and the condition will return.

The best advice, therefore, is to leave well alone and learn to live with the blemishes.

72
Fractures

A broken leg (*photo 1*) usually means that the horse has to be put down, not because the fracture cannot be repaired — in fact, advanced successful orthopaedic surgery is now practised in several equine hospitals and the techniques are likely to become increasingly efficient — but usually because it is not economical to operate, especially since there is only a slight chance of the horse being completely sound afterwards. Because of this, bad breaks are usually treated only in valuable stud stallions or brood mares.

There is, however, one type of fracture that can be treated successfully and comparatively inexpensively — a fracture without displacement (*photo 2*). Such a break should always be suspected when a horse has been kicked on the legs by another horse, especially when the kicker is shod. It is sometimes called a 'star' fracture, and in most cases can only be diagnosed by X-ray (*photo 3*). It is always advisable, therefore, to

2

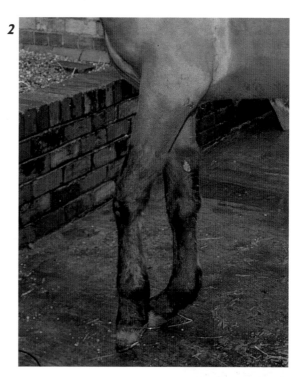

1

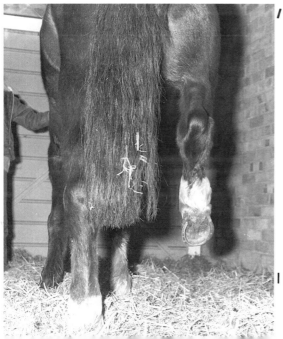

3

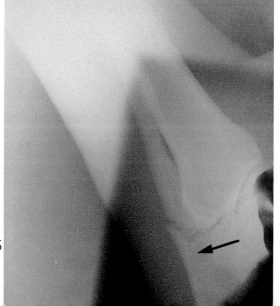

have a kicked leg X-rayed as quickly as possible. If the fracture is missed, it may displace later producing a compound break which will probably be irreparable.

Treatment

Obviously very much a job for your veterinary surgeon. He will most likely fit a plaster cast (*photo 4*). The patient may have to be slung and will certainly require at least six months' rest.

Because of the enforced inactivity, the diet should comprise only sloppy mashes and hay.

The prognosis is quite good, especially if the break does not impinge on a joint.

Split pastern

Another type of fracture well worth treating is a split pastern (*photo 5*). This can occur when jumping or turning sharply.

The case illustrated took three months to heal (*photo 6*).

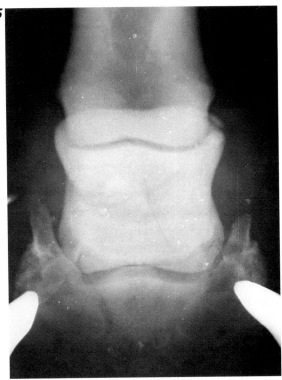

5

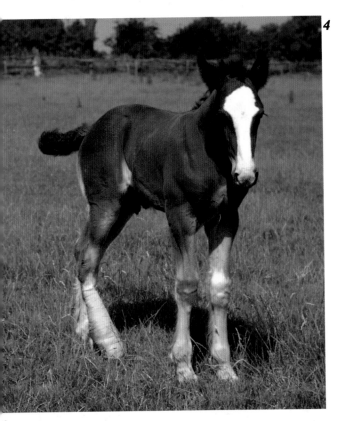

4

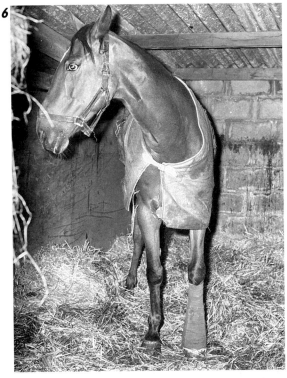

6

73
Curb

At the back of the hock there is a strong fibrous ligament which starts just below the point of the hock and runs down to the head of the metatarsus or cannon bone. The function of this ligament is largely to hold the bone of the point of the hock upwards; in other words, to anchor it in position.

In young horses, while galloping and jumping, this ligament may become strained — the strain is especially liable to happen in horses with bad conformation, e.g. 'sickle hocks'.

When the strain occurs the resultant swelling produces a 'curb' (*photo 1*).

Cause
Overwork, especially in young horses.

Symptoms
In the early stages there is, besides the swelling, considerable pain and usually slight lameness (*photo 2*). After two or three weeks the lameness and pain will subside, but the swelling or thickening remains. This thickening can be seen by standing back, or it can be felt by running the hand or the tips of the fingers from the point of the hock down the midline at the back (*photo 3*).

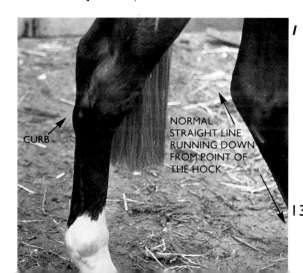

2

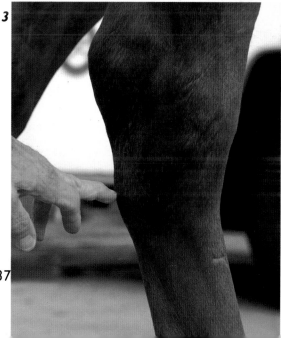

3

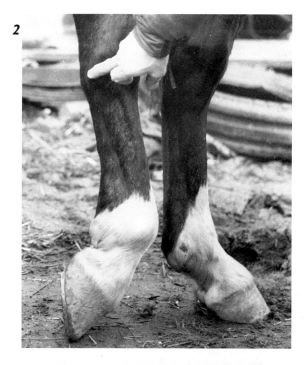

1

CURB

NORMAL STRAIGHT LINE RUNNING DOWN FROM POINT OF THE HOCK

137

Treatment

Complete rest for at least a fortnight, applying a cold hose to the part for five minutes, two or three times daily. **Don't** use liniments or blister, and if in the slightest doubt, consult your veterinary surgeon immediately.

If, at the end of fourteen days, the horse is sound he may be put into quiet, light work, but there should be no heavy work for at least three months. Overwork should be avoided at all times.

Is curb an unsoundness?

The answer is 'Yes' even though curb rarely recurs. Without doubt, it stands up better than any of the other tendon strains.

74
Sprain of the Suspensory Ligament

Sprain of the suspensory ligament is fortunately not very common. When it does happen, the part affected is usually the lower portion where the ligament branches near the fetlock (*photo 1*).

Cause

The suspensory ligaments are elastic ligaments which are involved in the support of the fetlock joint. Sprain or, in some cases, complete rupture can occur during fast galloping or jumping if the horse slips. In fact, it is safe to say that slipping during fast work or jumping is the primary cause.

Symptoms

Acute lameness, heat and pain immediately above the fetlock. If the ligament is ruptured, the fetlock will tend to drop down below its normal level even though it is still held by the superficial flexor tendon. Any injury to the suspensory ligament is serious and can take a long time to heal.

Treatment

Prolonged rest usually for at least the remainder of the season.

If the ligament branches are ruptured, then the fetlock must be supported either by elastic bandages or, in extreme cases, by a plaster cast.

Prognosis

A mild sprain often responds to a long rest and heals sufficiently for the horse to be raced sound. However, if the ligament is ruptured, complete healing is rare and treatment should only be considered in a mare or stallion which can be kept for breeding or stud.

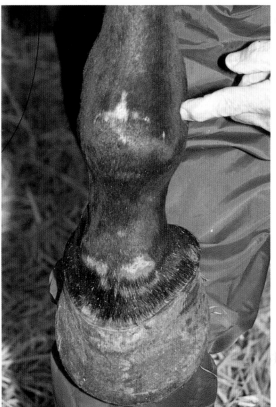

1

75
Stringhalt

This is a nervous condition.

Cause
Unknown.

Symptoms
An upward jerking of one or both hind legs due to an excessive flexion of the hock (*photo 1*). This is seen either when the horse walks or when he is turned sharply in a small circle (*photo 2*).

It is a non-painful condition and does not cause lameness. Nonetheless it is unsightly and constitutes a ***definite technical unsoundness***.

Many stringhalted horses are serviceable and gallop and jump perfectly satisfactorily. In fact, a stringhalted mare won the Grand National several years ago. Unfortunately the condition frequently gets worse with age.

Treatment
A surgical operation produces marked improvement in about 50 per cent of cases.

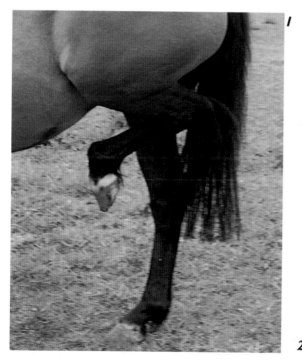

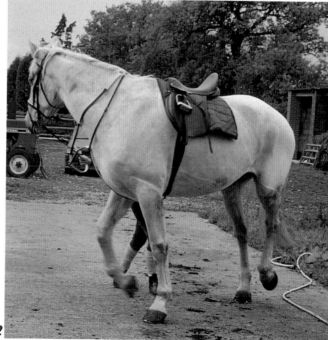

76
Shivering

This is another nervous disease, the cause of which is also unknown.

Symptoms

Involuntary shaking of certain groups of muscles, generally in the hind legs but occasionally in the fore.

When an affected animal is set or pushed backwards the tail rises and shivers (*photo 1*). During shoeing the symptoms may be exaggerated, especially when the shoe is being nailed on. The leg is pushed outwards, the shivering increases violently and the horse may almost fall onto his other side.

A drink of cold water or cold water thrown over a suspected leg will often make the symptoms more pronounced. Sometimes the horse refuses to allow a hind leg to be lifted

and this makes shoeing well-nigh impossible.

Treatment

There is no known cure for shivering but an intravenous or intramuscular injection of a tranquilliser will make the shoeing job much easier. Even the shiverer that refuses to lift a hind leg will relax sufficiently to do so comfortably.

Is it an unsoundness?

Yes, although, like stringhalt, it is a non-painful condition. Also, as with stringhalt, the shivering tends to get worse with age. Nonetheless, many shiverers can remain in steady hard work for a considerable number of years with the affliction apparently not spoiling their performance.

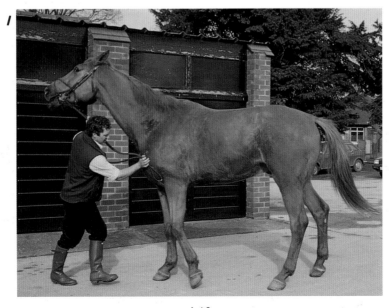

1

77
Lymphangitis
(Weed or Monday Morning Disease)

This is a condition which generally affects horses that are being heavily fed and hard worked. It flares up when they have to stop their active exercise suddenly, for instance, during spells of snow or frost. It is liable to occur, therefore, in hunters and in hard-working ponies.

Symptoms
The patient runs a high temperature — up to 105° or 106°F (40.5° or 41°C) — and an elevated pulse. There is a definite and often severe lameness of one leg, usually a hind leg (*photo 1*), but occasionally a fore.

The lymphatics, i.e. the drainage vessels in the leg, become swollen. On the inside and outside they can be felt like hard pencils with nodules along their course; these nodules are swollen lymphatic glands (*photo 2*).

Usually, when the swelling starts to appear, the pulse and temperature both drop to near normal despite the fact that the entire leg may continue to swell sometimes to almost twice the normal size.

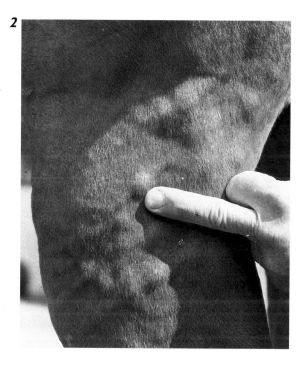

2

1

Treatment
Massage over the lymphatic glands and the swollen lymphatics with an ointment or an oily

liquid (*photo 3*). Continue the massage three or four times daily and combine each session with half an hour's forced exercise, provided,

of course, the patient is fit to walk (*photo 4*). Gentle exercise helps to get the lymphatics flowing freely again.

A laxative or light purgative will be given by your veterinary surgeon, and probably also a course of antibiotic injections to prevent secondary infection.

Prevention
When the horse is not at work its feed should be very much reduced and the oats cut out entirely.

3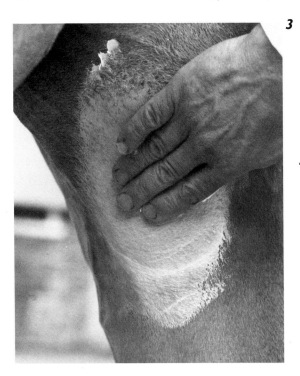

4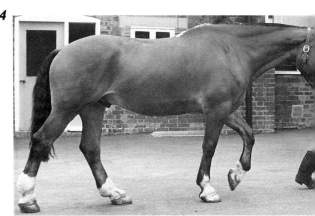

78
Ulcerative Lymphangitis (Canadian Pox)

This is an infectious skin disease, caused by the bacillus of pseudotuberculosis together with pus-producing bacteria like staphylococci and streptococci.

Small swellings which burst as abscesses

extend in lines up a fore or hind limb from an infected heel. The horse goes off its feed and runs a temperature. This condition is highly contagious and prompt veterinary attention and advice are vital.

79
Azoturia

Like lymphangitis, this is also a condition following idleness in fit horses. It occurs in hunters and racehorses that have had to be laid off work, usually because of the weather.

Symptoms

When exercise is started after the idle period, the animal will appear perfectly normal and may go for ten to thirty minutes before any signs are noticed. Stiffness is usually the first sign followed by sweating and obvious signs of pain from tensed-up hindquarters (*photo 1*).

The urine, if and when the patient stales, is coffee-coloured or reddish-brown, often described as 'wine-coloured'.

What happens is that a dysfunction of the lymphatics (drainage vessels) of the hind legs leads to a sort of muscular cramp.

The diagnostic 'wine-coloured' urine is *not* due to the presence of blood but to an excess of pigment.

Treatment

On no account must you attempt to walk the horse home. If you do, he will get progressively worse and will eventually go down and probably die.

Take him back to his stable in a horse box (*photo 2*) and send for your veterinary surgeon at once. He will inject antihistamine, cortisone or butazoladin and will order complete rest on a restricted diet.

There will be pain in the muscles of the loins but this will soon pass off with modern

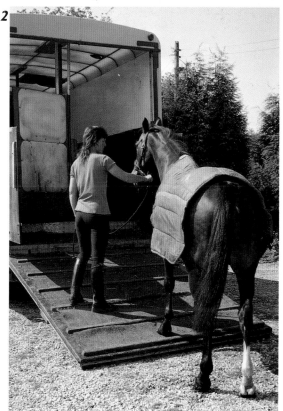

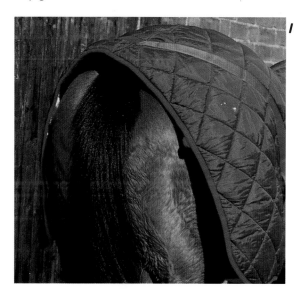

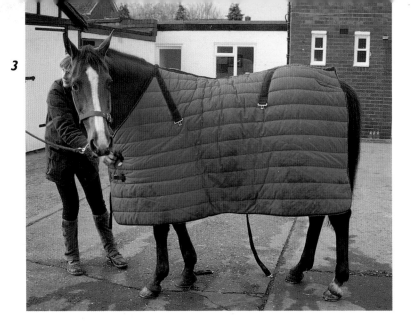

3

treatment. Nonetheless the old-fashioned treatment of hot blankets across the loins also helps considerably (*photo 3*).

Treated sensibly and promptly, most horses recover completely. If treatment is delayed, or if the horse is forced to continue after the onset of symptoms, death or permanent kidney damage may result.

If, after a day or two, the horse seems back to normal, then exercise can be resumed but this must be done very gently and very slowly. There is an old saying that still very much applies: 'When a horse is being exercised — walk the first mile, trot the next and do what the hell you like after that.'

Prevention

When the horse is not at exercise, drastically reduce the feed and cut out oats entirely.

Set-fast

Set-fast is a mild form of azoturia seen mostly in young racehorses, yearlings or two-year-olds which are being worked excessively.

Symptoms

The colt or filly stiffens up across the back after exercise and runs a temperature of around 104-105°F (40-40.5°C).

Treatment

The same as for azoturia with rest, a laxative diet and a gradual return to work the most important factors.

Prevention

Grade the feeding carefully according to the work done and bring on the youngsters with careful progression in the training.

80
Rigged Back

A horse is said to have 'rigged' his back when he partially loses control of his hindquarters (*photo 1*).

Cause

A fall during jumping or hunting. 'Rigged back' used to be a major danger when horses had to be cast for operations. Nowadays intravenous anaesthetics have virtually eliminated the risk. The injury is undoubtedly a partial or complete displacement of a spinal (intravertebral) disc, though some scientists dispute this.

Treatment
The condition is incurable, though prolonged rest at pasture may be tried.

Just occasionally a 'rigged back' syndrome can be produced by a fibrositis or by a direct injury to the back. Such cases require skilled attention and special nursing combined with prolonged rest.

The so-called 'cold back' reaction seen occasionally when a horse is saddled up is usually due to muscular pain and can be treated satisfactorily with butazolodin and good management.

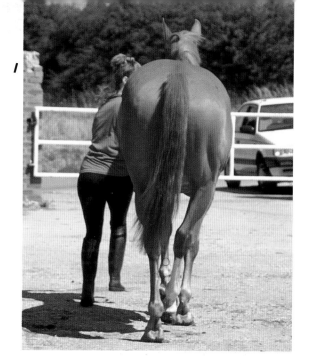

81
Pelvic Lameness

Pelvic lameness is difficult to diagnose, but fortunately is uncommon.

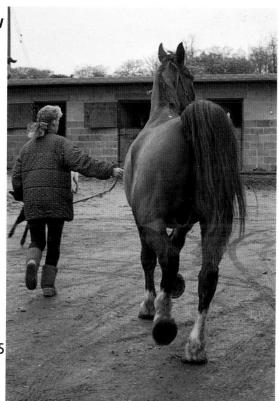

Cause
Invariably an injury such as falling on a hard road (*photo 1*), especially in the heavier breeds. A similar type of lameness in a grey horse can be caused by internal pressure on the pelvis from a melanoma.

Symptoms
Marked lameness in the hind leg or legs, usually unilateral but sometimes bilateral.

Treatment
Prolonged rest.

Prognosis
Very poor.

82
Grass Humor

Occasionally, a horse may be brought up from grass with one or all four legs markedly swollen (*photo 1*). The swelling is oedematous or dropsical, and there may be a slight serous discharge from the skin surface, but the horse or pony is rarely lame.

This is the condition known in many parts of the country as 'grass humor'.

Symptoms
The outstanding symptom is that the swelling is reasonably soft and pits on pressure (*photo 2*).

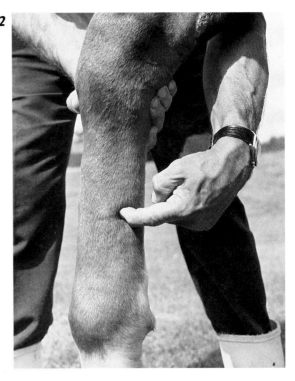

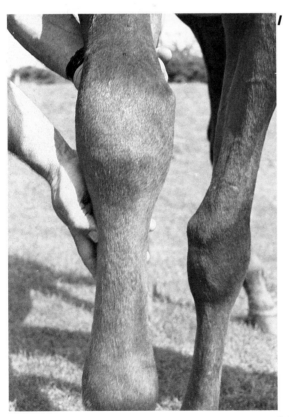

What causes it?
Since the cause is often obscure, grass humor is described as an allergic condition. It is probably triggered off by nettle rash or by the stings of wasps, bees or other flies or insects.

Treatment
Hot and cold fomentations may be tried, but as a rule the swelling disappears with exercise. It is rarely serious unless attended by lameness. Nonetheless veterinary surgeons have modern antihistamine and diuretic injections which will remove the swellings quickly and, in any case, it is much better to consult them if only to confirm the diagnosis.

83
Grease

This is a condition seen comparatively rarely in hunters and ponies. It was a common sight among the heavy draft Shires and Clydesdales, particularly Shires, when they were widely used. Nowadays I think it fair to say that it is likely to occur only in heavyweight hunters that have been bred from draft mares (*photo 1*).

Cause
Too much food in relation to exercise or work done. Grease often follows repeated attacks of lymphangitis.

Symptoms
The term 'grease' vividly describes the condition. The leg — usually one but sometimes both of the hind ones — swells up and exudes a foul-smelling greasy discharge (*photo 2*). Lameness is not usually present except when the condition is complicated by infection.

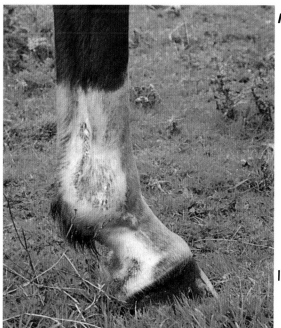

2

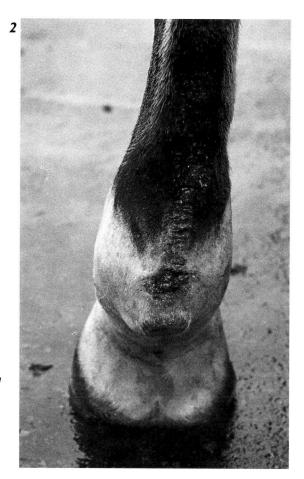

1

Treatment
Stop feeding nuts, oats or linseed. Give only good hay and a bran mash twice daily. Get the animal into regular work and house in a roomy loose box.

The golden rule is: '**Never** apply grease to a greasy surface' — so all ointments or creams are contra-indicated.

Wash with soap and water, dry thoroughly

147

and apply a lotion (*photo 3*) comprising:
  zinc sulphate — 15g (½ oz)
  lead acetate — 7.5g (¼ oz)
  water — 1 litre (1½ pints)

If an infection is present, an antibiotic aerosol containing chloramphenicol and gentian violet is the best dressing. Some horses violently resent aerosols. In such cases, the antibiotics have to be applied in lotion form.

Prevention
Feed strictly according to work done and never keep a heavyweight hunter standing idle in a box or stable.

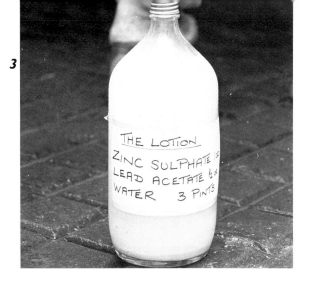

3

THE LOTION
ZINC SULPHATE 15
LEAD ACETATE ¼
WATER 3 PINTS

84
Mud Fever

Another condition in many ways similar to grease is mud fever (*photo 1*).

Cause
Bad management, which allows repeated

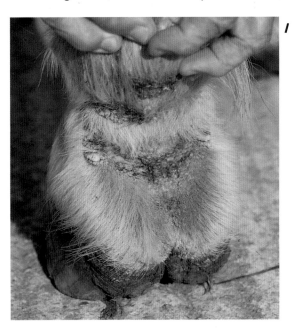

1

immersion of the legs in mud. The hardened mud, especially when it freezes, produces an irritation and thickening of the skin surface. ***Mud fever is not caused by a bug and is not contagious, though occasionally in severe cases a fungus called Dermatophilus congolensis may complicate the picture.***

Treatment
Wash the mud off thoroughly with hot water and soap flakes; dry carefully and apply zinc sulphate and lead acetate lotion made up as for grease once daily.

Vaseline and other emollient dressings containing oil or lanolin may also be used; they are much more effective than some of the modern synthetic creams.

Prevention
Leave the legs unclipped during the hunting season and coat them with petroleum jelly before each outing.

Wash and dry the legs thoroughly whenever necessary.

Feet

85
The Horse's Foot: General Anatomy

A simple knowledge of the anatomy and physiology of the horse's foot helps tremendously in understanding the need for care and also the various conditions and problems that can arise.

The coronary band
It is from the coronary band that all the horn grows. The horn grows downwards (*photo 1*).

The frog
The frog (*photo 2*) helps to pump the blood through the hoof. It also acts as a cushion to absorb concussion. The frog doesn't bruise easily and certainly not as easily as the sole.

The navicular bone and the pedal bone
The navicular bone acts as a wedge to guide the tendons over onto the pedal bone and

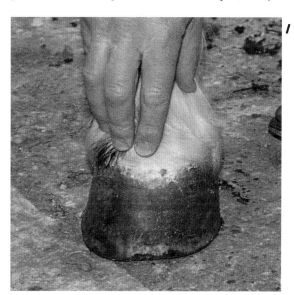

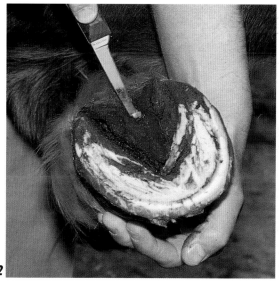

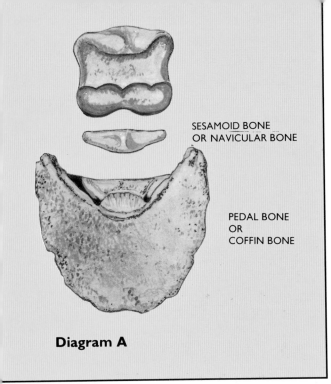

SESAMOID BONE
OR NAVICULAR BONE

PEDAL BONE
OR
COFFIN BONE

Diagram A

Diagram B

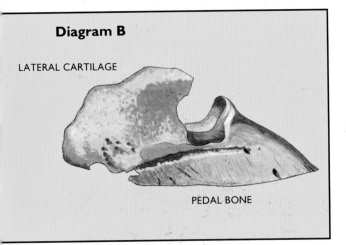

LATERAL CARTILAGE

PEDAL BONE

Diagram C

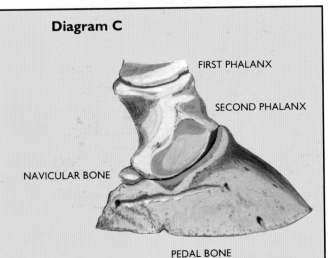

FIRST PHALANX

SECOND PHALANX

NAVICULAR BONE

PEDAL BONE

keeps the tendons moving freely (*see diagram A*). Needless to say, though small, the navicular bone is very important and if anything goes wrong with it the results are serious (see 'Navicular Disease', page 162).

The pedal bone is the main bone of the foot and is shaped approximately like the foot in miniature.

The lateral cartilage
The lateral cartilage forms a wing on either side of the pedal bone (*see diagram B*).

The second phalanx
The second phalanx fits into the articular surface of the pedal bone, with the navicular bone fitting in behind (*see diagram C*).

The sole and the wall
The sole covers over and protects the solar surface of the sensitive laminae and the pedal bone. The wall protects the lateral aspects of both.

The white line
This is the junction of the wall and the sole and is clearly visible as a white line following the circumference of the wall (*photo 3*).

3

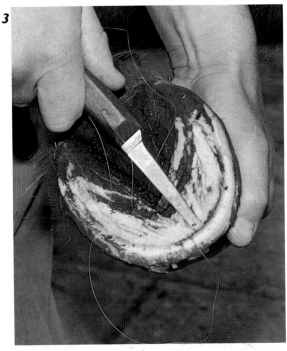

86
Bruised Sole

The sole has no sensation on its own but it bruises very easily, in some breeds more readily than in others. For example, the Arab has a very hard sole, whereas the thoroughbred is much more bruise-prone.

Cause
Neglect leading to overgrowth of horn so that the sole surface becomes flat or convex instead of concave; jumping on stone or other hard objects; backing or galloping over stony roads.

Symptoms
Marked lameness. The horse flinches when the sole is tapped with a hammer or the foot is compressed with blacksmith's pincers. When the sole is scrubbed with hot water and washing soda the bruise may be apparent, but usually to identify the spot it is necessary to remove the shoe and pare off the superficial layer of the sole.

Treatment
If not already done, remove the shoe (*photo 1*) and pare out the entire bruised area so that it is free from pressure (*photo 2*); poultice and rest for at least a week.

Thereafter, if anxious to get the horse back to work, the sole can be dressed with stockholm tar and the foot can be shod with a 'leather'. The best material to use is balata belting; this may be difficult to procure, though the broad belts from old belting machines are usually made of this material, and if they are no longer in use on the machine, may be cut up as protective soles when they are required.

1

2

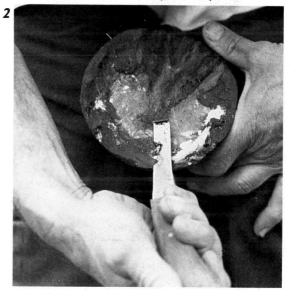

Special protective pads can be bought (*photo 3*).

Prevention

Simple commonsense — regular shoeing and the routine use of the hoof-pick (*photo 4*), together with the avoidance of stony lanes during exercise or work.

Really severe bruising often occurs in the flat soles of the pony or horse which has suffered one or several attacks of laminitis. The laminae become extended from the wall and if the shoes are left on too long bruising becomes extensive and acutely painful causing marked lameness (*photo 5*).

Such cases should be shod **once a month** with the special broad-webbed seated out shoes (*photo 6*) recommended for chronic laminitis (page 169).

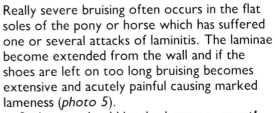

3

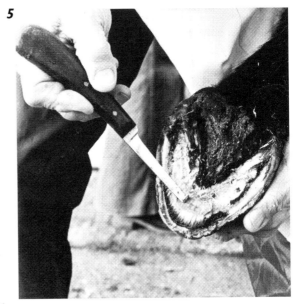

5

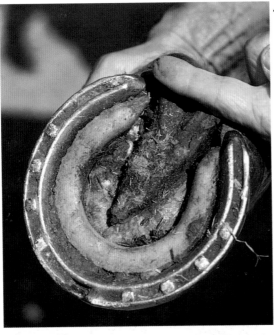

4

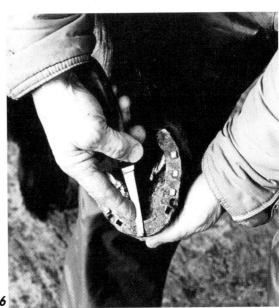

6

87
Corns

A corn is simply bruising of the sole in the sharp angle between the wall and the heel (*photo 1*).

Cause
Often associated with either bad shoeing or the shoes being left on too long.

Symptoms
Lameness. Many a so-called 'recurring and mysterious lameness' has proved, on careful searching of the feet, to be due to a simple corn.

Treatment
This is a job for the veterinary surgeon or blacksmith. The shoes have to be removed and the bruised area completely cut out.

Thereafter the shoe can be put on again but this time with a widened webb at the appropriate heel to give protection to the corn area without exerting any pressure.

General care of the foot
The routine is simple and comprises regular dressing; regular shoeing; conscientious use of the hoof-pick; daily painting with hoof oil (*photo 2*) when stabled or at work. The oil not only makes the foot look better but some of it penetrates the wall. It keeps the wall soft, and helps to prevent cracks (see 'Grass Cracks' and 'Sand Cracks', pp 157 & 158).

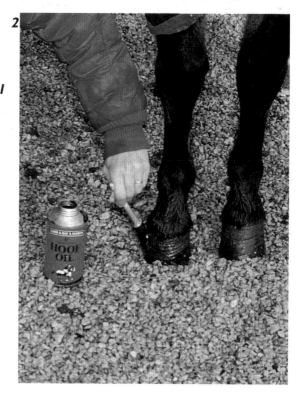

2

1

88
Picked-up Nails and Suppurating Feet

When at college, again and again we were told by our Professor: 'It does not matter where you think a horse is lame, always test the foot.' This has proved to be probably the soundest advice of all in horse veterinary practice.

Naturally enough, a horse or pony is always liable to 'pick up' a nail or to tramp on a sharp piece of metal, stone, glass or wood — and if any of these foreign objects penetrate the sole to the sensitive structure underneath, then subsequent suppuration is a near certainty.

A common place to find a picked-up nail is at or near the point of the frog. The reason for this is simple — the nail gets turned up by the toe, it then slides along the sole until it catches against the frog where it penetrates.

Symptoms

If the sensitive structures are damaged badly, then marked lameness is apparent immediately.

In most cases, however, lameness does not appear for several days. The reason for this is that it is usually four, five or even six or seven days before the infective material, carried in by the nail, produces suppuration, with pus and abscess formation. This causes acute pressure on the sensitive areas and this in turn provides lameness, which is often very severe indeed, causing the horse to sweat and paw continually at the ground.

In the early stages, however, the first symptom is usually just pronounced lameness.

When the wall of the affected foot is tapped with a hammer (*photo 1*), the horse will pick the foot up sharply and will often move it up and down and shiver, thus showing clear evidence of pain. The same will happen when the sole is tapped or squeezed between

the jaws of a pair of blacksmith's pincers (*photo 2*). In fact, when searching for the

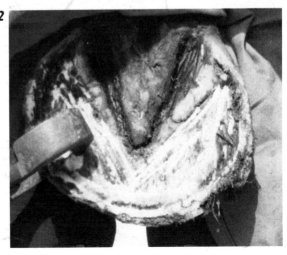

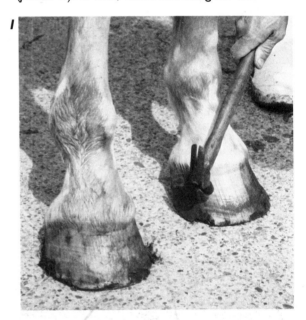

abscess the veterinary surgeon will often be able to localise the infected area by tapping with the hammer or squeezing with the pincers.

Treatment

Send for your veterinary surgeon immediately. If a nail is present, pull it out but note carefully the spot, to assist the veterinary surgeon when he arrives. Some veterinary surgeons will arrange to have a blacksmith in attendance to remove the shoe and do the cutting out under supervision. Others prefer to do the job on their own.

The main point will be the thorough opening up of the focus of infection to ensure complete drainage (*photo 3*). Again and again the advice of the experienced veterinary surgeon is: 'The bigger the hole you cut out, the quicker the horse will recover.'

If the abscess is not opened up fairly promptly, the pus will take the line of least resistance and the infection will spread either between the sensitive laminae and sole, or between the sensitive laminae and wall. If, of course, it follows the latter course, it may burst at the top of the hoof causing prolonged lameness and the possibility of bone infection. Prompt and efficient drainage is therefore vital.

After the pus has poured out, the cavity should be syringed out with antibiotic or antiseptic (*photo 4*).

Subsequently, the foot should be soaked in hot water containing antiseptic twice daily (*photo 5*) and covered over with a clean sack to prevent the drainage hole being blocked by dirt.

4
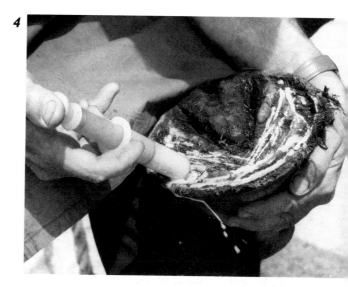

5
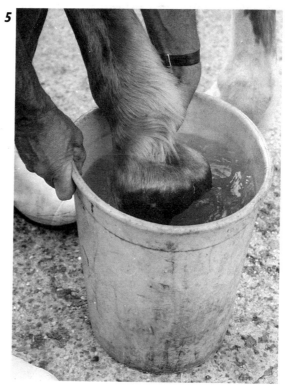

3

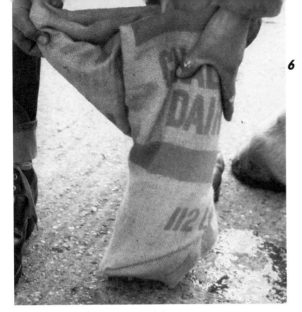

6

Poulticing can be useful (*photo 6*), but if a bran poultice is used, a non-irritant antiseptic must be mixed with the bran, and the poultice should be renewed night and morning taking care to remove all the bran from the hole each time. Obviously, if poulticing is not done conscientiously, the sole object of effective drainage will be defeated. Personally I prefer the twice-daily soaking method.

Another vital treatment — an injection against tetanus (*photo 7*). Even if the horse has been inoculated against tetanus, a booster dose of tetanus antitoxin is advisable since the punctured wound in the foot provides the ideal conditions for the growth of the tetanus germs and also because a wound on the sole of the foot is much more likely to be contaminated by tetanus spores than a wound anywhere else on the body.

After five or six days' treatment, provided the horse is sound and all trace of pus has disappeared, the hole can be packed with stockholm tar and cotton wool, or tow, and the shoe can be replaced with a 'leather' underneath, covering the entire sole area (*photos 8 & 9*).

The leather should be left on for at least a week to ten days. Then, if still no signs of lameness, it can be removed by running a sharp knife round the inside of the shoe or by re-shoeing.

7

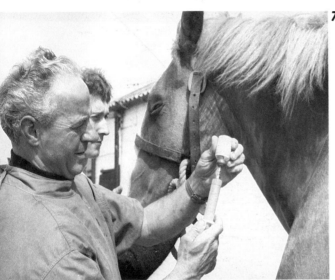

9

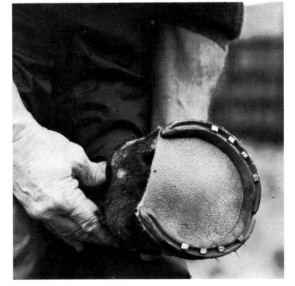

8

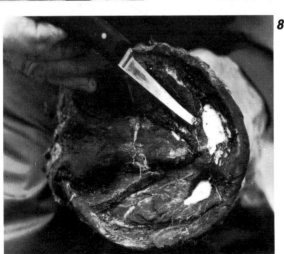

89
Grass Cracks

Grass cracks occur when the horse or pony is turned out at grass without shoes.

They are characterised by the fact that they start at the ground surface and extend or split in an upward direction (*photos 1 & 2*). Sand cracks, on the other hand, start at the hoof head and spread downwards (see page 158).

Treatment
Get the blacksmith to dress the hoof if the cracks are very bad. In consultation with the veterinary surgeon he will probably shoe the horse with a clip on each side of the crack. This is usually all that is necessary because with ordinary grass cracks the hooves grow down and the crack eventually disappears.

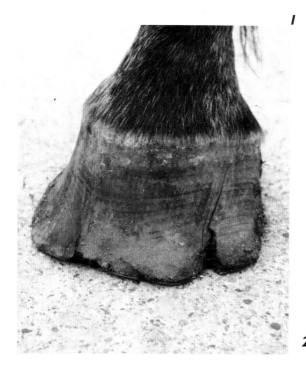

2

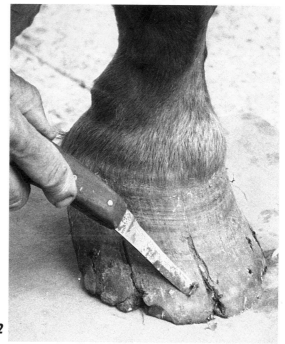

1

90
Sand Cracks

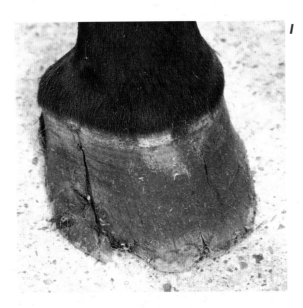

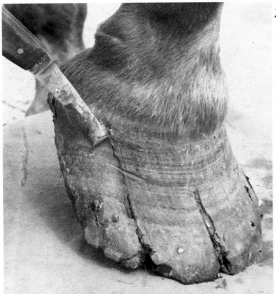

1 These are much more serious than grass cracks and require veterinary attention. Sand cracks are distinguished by the fact that they grow or extend downwards from the top of the hoof (*photos 1 & 2*), causing pain and lameness.

Cause

Sand cracks are usually caused by an injury to the coronary band — the band at the top of the hoof from which all horn growth emanates.

Treatment

Invariably the treatment of sand cracks calls for the supervision of a veterinary surgeon. He will probably advise firing the crack and shoeing with clips each side of the crack. He may or may not recommend stimulant applications to the coronary band.

2 If the crack is not too extensive, in order to prevent the persistent stress on the coronary band and to avoid the sensitive laminae under the wall being pinched between the edges of the crack, the veterinary surgeon may anaesthetise the horse and remove a triangular piece of the wall with the apex of the triangle at the lowest extremity of the crack and the base of the triangle at the coronary band. This will enable the coronet to secrete new horn to fill the gap and will considerably alleviate the lameness.

It is important to remember that sand cracks can only be kept in control by the combined efforts of the veterinary surgeon and blacksmith, and this means that local treatments are not only a waste of time and money, but may well jeopardise the future soundness of the horse.

91
Cracked Heels

The term 'cracked heel' is a slight misnomer because the condition occurs not actually in the heel but usually in the hollow of the pastern.

Cracked heels (*photo 1*) are found usually in horses or ponies wintered out on soaking wet pastures and mud. They also occur in horses where the legs are washed repeatedly, instead of being brushed, and not dried properly.

Symptoms
The condition starts with scurf and scabs which come off, leaving nasty painful cracks (*photo 2*) which, if not treated promptly, become infected.

The horse may or may not be lame depending on how long the cracks have been there.

Treatment
Wash all the scurf and scabs off with soap and water and then dry *very* thoroughly (*photo 3*).

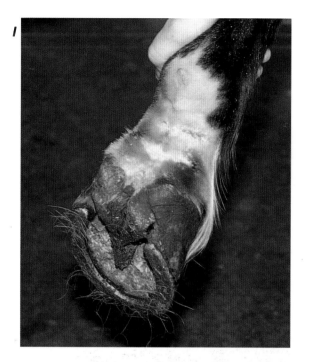

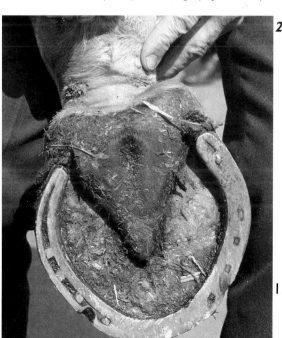

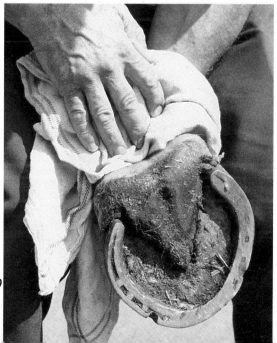

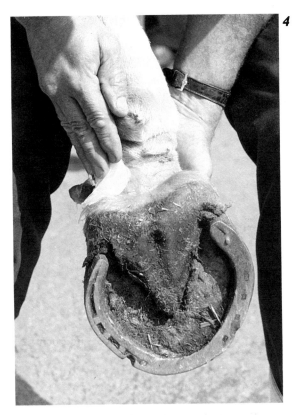

4   Apply either Vaseline or any reputable healing and antiseptic ointment, such as the old-fashioned Lasser's paste or calamine ointment (*photo 4*). I have found a proprietary preparation called Storaxyl very satisfactory.

Dry powder is contra-indicated and should never be used, since it makes the cracks worse. Drying and hardening aerosols also have this adverse effect and should be avoided.

Cortisone creams and ointments are also contra-indicated because, though they may allay any inflammation, they prevent healing.

If the horse or pony is lame, it must be rested (*photo 5*). If the condition has been caught early and the patient is not lame, confine him to light exercise only until treatment is complete.

Prevention

When the horse or pony is out on wet muddy pastures, a protective smear of vaseline over the hollow of the pastern at fairly regular intervals will prevent cracking (*photo 6*). A twice-weekly dressing should be sufficient.

If the weather and pastures are dry the protective Vaseline dressing is not necessary.

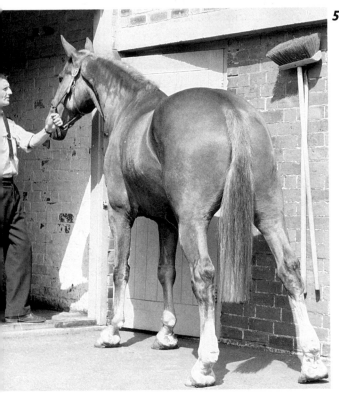

5

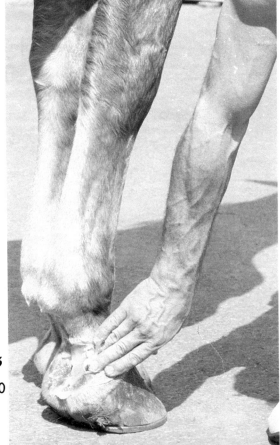

6

160

92
Quittor

In the chapter on sidebones (see page 170) there is a simple explanation as to what the lateral cartilages are and where they are situated.

Occasionally, as a result of an injury in the area, part of a lateral cartilage dies. When this happens, a tract of pus travels up towards the hoof-head or coronet and breaks out, producing a fistula leading directly down to the dead portion of cartilage (*photo 1*).

The condition is unmistakable and invariably the horse is very lame.

Treatment
The only treatment is surgery and this should be done by your veterinary surgeon at the earliest possible moment, to avoid involvement of the nearby tendons and bone.

Surgery comprises dissecting down to the damaged cartilage and actually cutting out the dead portion (*photo 2*).

The resultant wound is then filled with antibiotics or sulpha drugs and bandaged up firmly.

The prognosis is quite good provided the operation is performed without delay.

1

2

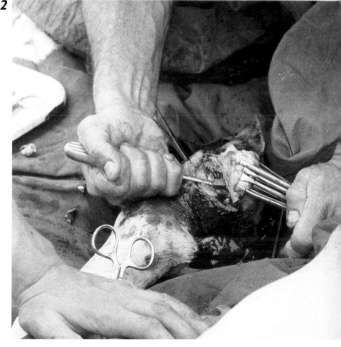

93
Navicular Disease

Navicular disease can occur in horses or ponies of any age, but it is most commonly seen in older animals and often in those that have had a fair amount of percussion on their forefeet during life, e.g. through road work or show-jumping (*photo 1*). When it appears in young horses it can be hereditary. But often it is caused by premature hard work.

It has been my experience that wherever you have a persistent obscure lameness in the fore end, the most likely cause is navicular disease.

What is the condition?
Navicular disease is a disease of the navicular bone (*see diagram*), a thin, elongated bone at the back of the foot. It lies across the pedal bone and between it and the second phalanx, acting more or less as a wedge but forming part of the joint.

Over the navicular bone's posterior, or rear extremity, runs a flexor tendon.

When the disease — a rarefying ostitis — attacks the bone it eats into it, generally on the rear surface, causing hollows and cavities to appear; these are called lacunae. Naturally, this disintegration of the bone produces a chronic and persistent pain.

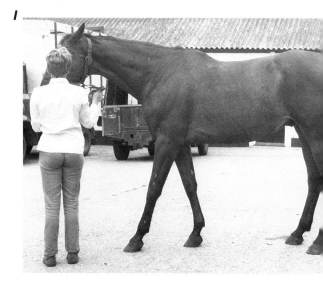

Which feet does it affect?
It is much more common in the forefeet (*photo 2*); in fact, it is rare in the hind. Generally speaking, both forefeet are affected simultaneously. This means that, in the early stages, lameness may not be noticed simply because it is equal in both forelegs.

Symptoms
As already stated, any persistent obscure lameness in the forelegs should always be regarded as a suspect navicular disease.

The typical 'navicular gait' is almost diagnostic. The horse becomes 'pottery', that is, he does not extend his forefeet in the normal way but goes with short steps, putting his toes down first in a simple attempt to keep his weight off the heels (*photo 3*).

An examination of the shoes of a navicular horse will show that the toes are much more worn than the heels (*photo 4*).

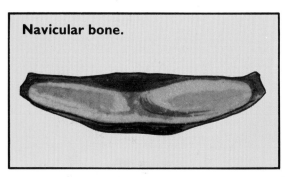

Navicular bone.

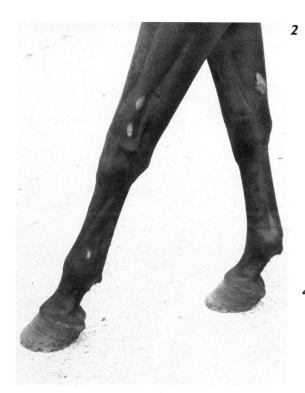

2

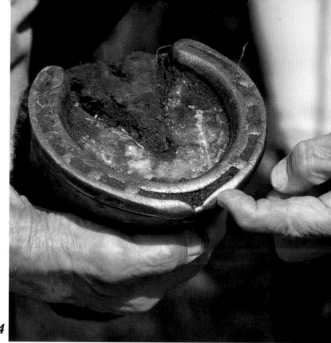

4

There is also a tendency to stumble, but both the stumbling and pottering are usually more apparent either when the horse is first brought out of the stable or when the horse is trotted downhill, with the weight being thrown on the front end (*photo 5*).

3

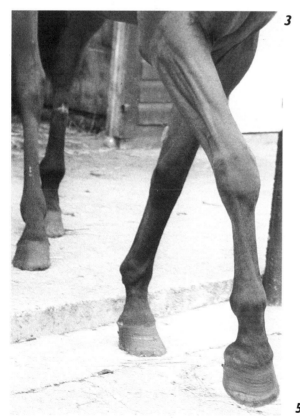

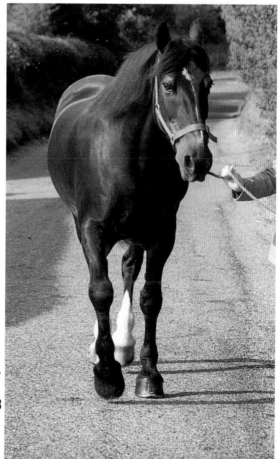

5

163

As the disease develops, the hoof first becomes contracted, then what we term 'boxey' — the walls become more vertical and the heels straight and deep, rather like a mule's or a donkey's foot. The sole becomes abnormally concave (*photo 6*).

Diagnosis
The tentative diagnosis can be made with confidence on the symptoms, but positive confirmation is possible only by X-ray (*photo 7*).

Before X-raying the foot the veterinary surgeon will probably block the nerves to the foot with local anaesthetic, thereby locating the pain and trouble with certainty (*photo 8*).

The X-ray can reveal the disease in an early stage by showing the lacunae. Also, at each end of the bone a little growth or 'spur'

6
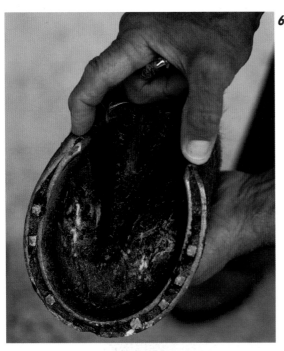

8
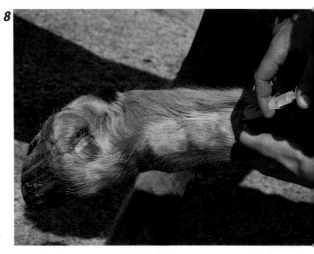

7
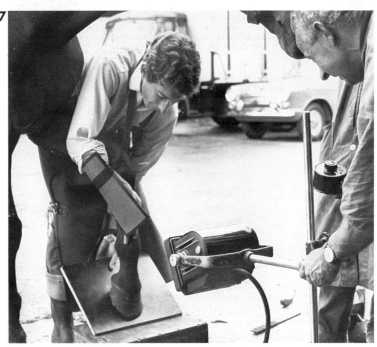

frequently appears (*photo 9*).

Treatment
There is no known cure, but a neurectomy operation (cutting the nerves that supply the sensation to the area) may give full usefulness and satisfaction for many years (*photo 10*). It certainly removes all pain immediately. Neurectomy is not a 'cure' — it is merely a means of alleviating the pain and thereby stopping the lameness.

After neurectomy (often called 'denerving') careful shoeing and daily examination of the feet must be carried out or better still the patient should be shod with a leather (see page 156). Should the horse pick up a nail or be pricked when shoeing, then sepsis will set in and it may not be noticed until the sole or wall is extensively under-run (*photo 11*). This, of course, is what produces the anti-denerving tales of hooves dropping off after the operation.

It is my opinion that neurectomy can always be embarked on with confidence provided the owner will assiduously undertake to watch the feet.

A drug called butazoldin, marketed under several proprietary names, is most effective in early cases of navicular disease and will often keep the horse sound for long periods. However, the drug has to be given daily and continually. It does nothing to cure or halt the disease: it merely alleviates the pain and increases the horse's useful life. I do not hesitate to prescribe it and certainly do not advocate neurectomy until after the butazoldin has lost its effect.

9

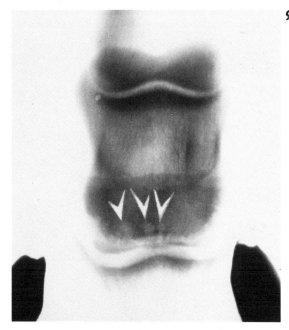

11

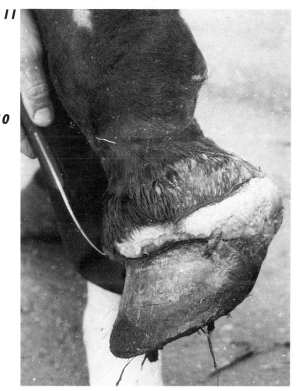

10

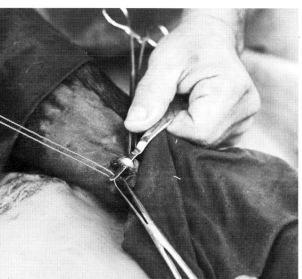

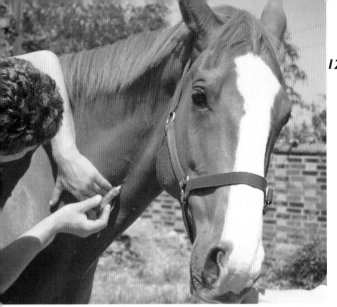

12   The butazoldin powders can be given in the food once or twice daily.

When examining a horse for soundness, a veterinary surgeon should always bloodtest for butazoldin, which may be masking an obscure lameness (*photo 12*).

Some experiments at the Equine Research Centre in Newmarket have raised hope for a satisfactory treatment. This comprises the controlled use of warfarin, which prolongs the time the blood takes to clot, thereby preventing further blood clots in the arteries supplying the navicular bone.

It is blood clotting — that is, arterial thrombosis — that produces the typical lacunae.

94
Laminitis

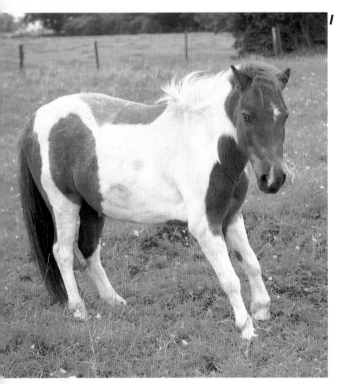

1   Laminitis is a condition affecting the feet of horses, usually the forefeet (*photo 1*).

The term 'laminitis' simply means an inflammation of laminae. The junction between the horny hoof and the pedal bone (which forms the centre of the foot) is made by the sensitive laminae (*see diagram*). The laminae from the hoof and the laminae from the bone dovetail, rather like paper-thin cogs of two

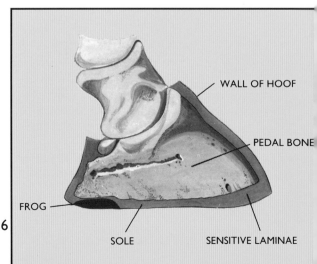

WALL OF HOOF

PEDAL BONE

FROG

SENSITIVE LAMINAE

SOLE

minute wheels. When these laminae become inflamed, then the condition is laminitis.

As with all inflammations, there occurs swelling — but because of the firm wall of the hoof and sole, there is no room for the swelling and this leads to very acute pain.

Causes

There are several causes:

1. Fat animals eating too much grass and taking very little exercise. It has been my experience that this is by far the commonest cause, especially when the grass contains a high percentage of rich young clover (*photo 2*).

2. Feeding too much grain or corn.

3. An allergy.

4. A portion of retained afterbirth in a mare.

5. Standing for excessively long periods — for instance, when travelling in railway wagons or boats.

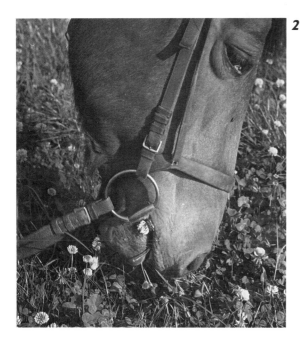

2

Symptoms

In acute laminitis the temperature rises slightly — one or two degrees — but the pulse rises considerably.

There is very marked lameness, heat round the coronet, and obvious pain when the foot is tapped with a knife handle or a hammer.

The lameness is in the two front feet; when the horse is asked to move he arches his back, stretches his head out in front of him and pushes his hind legs underneath in an attempt to take the weight off the forefeet (*photo 3*).

He has difficulty in lying down and in getting up — so when he does go down he will lie, often flat out on his side, for abnormally long periods (*photo 4*).

If the acute inflammation is prolonged for any length of time, the laminae between the horn and the bone become detached. The weight of the horse then causes the pedal bone

3

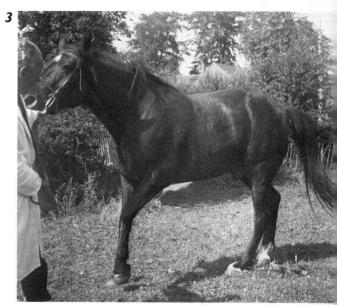

4

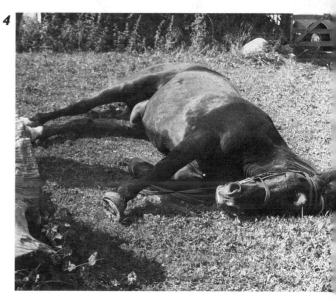

to sink downwards (*photo 5*) so that the sole becomes flat instead of concave, or it may even become convex and press on the ground (*photo 6*).

Also, with the bone sinking, the horny hoof, instead of being straight from the coronary band to the solar surface, becomes concave and deep ridges appear around the hoof (*photo 7*).

All this produces what is recognised as **chronic** laminitis.

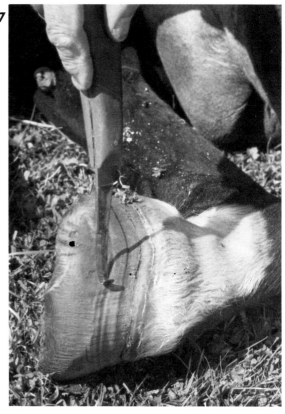

7

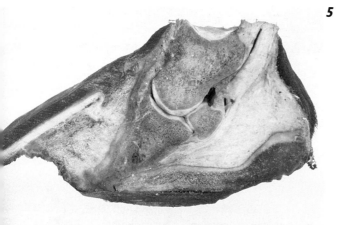

5

6

Treatment

There is no real specific treatment, but cortisone and antihistamine injections, promptly given, can reduce the inflammation rapidly and do much to prevent the 'dropped sole'. So it is vitally important to call the veterinary surgeon immediately.

The cause must be ascertained and rectified at once. For example, if due to over-feeding, the horse must be dieted on the lightest possible diet.

The front shoes should be removed (*photo 8*).

If the pony or horse is at grass, he should be housed in a spacious loose box well bedded down with peat moss or sawdust, and ample fresh drinking water should be provided. He should be fed only rationed good-quality hay and exercised on a halter three times a day. When apparently better he can be grazed for no more than *one* hour daily on a bare pasture.

Local treatment such as cold hosing from the fetlocks downwards three or four times a day (*photo 9*), or standing the horse in a cold running brook for several half-hour periods during the day, can be very helpful. A cold wet clay poultice, kept cold and wet by pouring water over it, is also effective.

Chronic cases require special (broad-webbed seated out) surgical shoes which should be made under veterinary supervision and fitted hot; they should be renewed at least once a month.

Prevention

Prevention is far better than having to treat laminitis and is quite simple. Avoid all the likely causes — if a mare holds her afterbirth, have her attended to at once.

Never over-feed and do not leave fat ponies to gorge themselves on rich pastures. A novel but effective way to control over-eating is to muzzle the pony when it is being exercised at pasture (*photo 10*). The muzzle does not interfere with drinking.

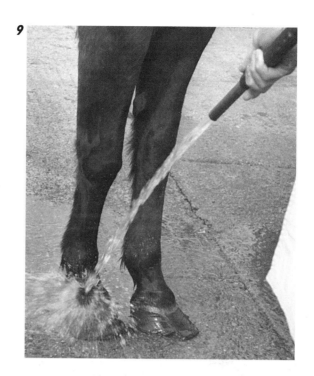

9

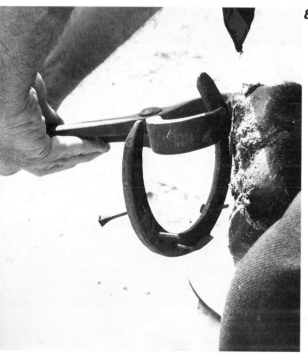

8

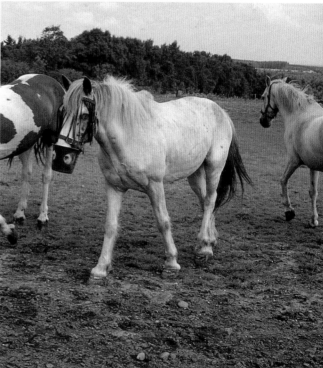

10

95
Pedal Ostitis

Pedal ostitis (inflammation of the pedal bone) is caused by excessive percussion on hard roads or by injury. It produces callus formation or defective growth of any part of the pedal bone, and the subsequent increased pressure within the hoof causes marked lameness. The condition can only be diagnosed by X-ray.

Treatment
Like navicular disease, pedal ostitis is very difficult to treat. Butazolidin may give some relief. Denerving may be the only answer, but I have had considerable success by grooving the wall of the hoof to relieve the pressure (*photo 1*). Certainly this is well worth trying before resorting to denerving.

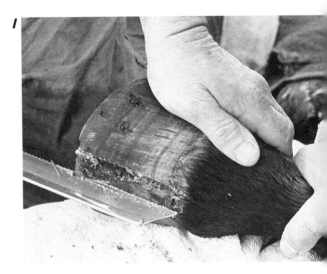

96
Sidebones

Contrary to what many people think and say, sidebones are not hereditary.

Once again some knowledge of simple anatomy is required to understand exactly what a sidebone is.

At the side of each pedal bone (the lowest bone of the foot) — both the inside and outside — there is a wing of cartilage called the lateral cartilage (*see diagram*).

Frequently in heavy horses, but rarely in the lighter breeds and ponies, this cartilage changes into bone. When this happens the resultant hard lump of bone is called a sidebone (*photos 1 & 2*).

Cause
In the heavy horses the ossification often occurs spontaneously for no apparent reason, but in light horses or ponies the cause is usually an injury of some sort.

Lateral Cartilage

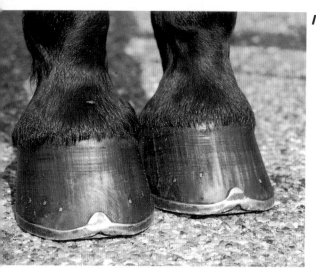

LATERAL CARTILAGE

attempting to flex or bend inward the cartilage.

Are they an unsoundness?
Sidebones can never be considered to constitute a serious condition. Nonetheless they *are* an unsoundness and a horse should never be bought or sold as sound if any sidebone formation exists.

Prognosis
Many heavy horses have gone through the whole of their working life with sidebones and have never ever shown any signs of lameness.

Treatment
As with pedal ostitis, where lameness is present, a surgical treatment worth trying comprises sawing the wall of the hoof to spread or 'splay' it. This often allays the laming effect of the tightness in the tissues around the sidebone (*photo 3*).

However I have found that the only apparent permanent cure for sidebone lameness is the bold surgery of cutting out the offending sidebones.

The horse is given a general anaesthetic and

1

3

2

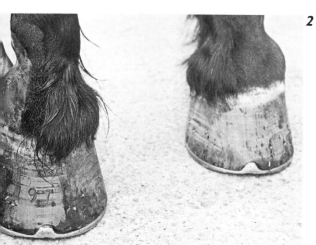

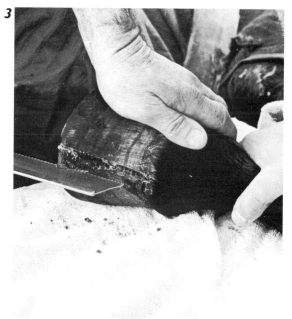

Symptoms
Lameness is negligible or completely absent. The hard bone formation can be felt by

the operation site is clipped, shaved and thoroughly sterilised (*photo 4*).

The lateral cartilage is then exposed by careful dissection and the offending sidebone is chiselled out (*photo 5*).

A modern sulpha and antibiotic dressing ensures rapid and uncomplicated healing.

5

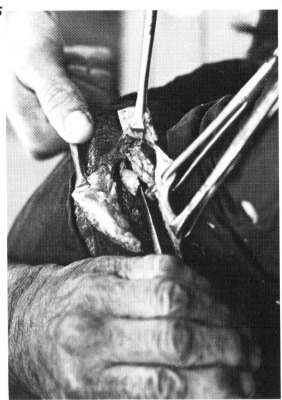

4

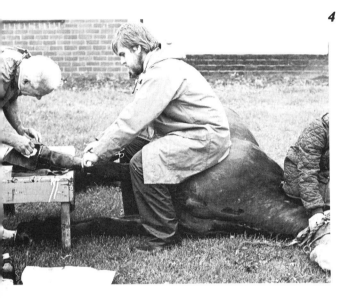

97
Seedy Toe

Seedy toe is a separation of the wall of the hoof from the sensitive laminae (commonly called the 'quick') (*photo 1*).

Cause
A seedy toe can start with a slight crack or injury between the sole and the wall. Gradually dirt may work into the cavity and eventually produce a seedy toe.

The most common cause, however, is foot neglect. In fact, seedy toe could be said to be a frequent complication of lack of foot care. What happens is that the overgrown wall is pushed away from the soft tissues by the

1

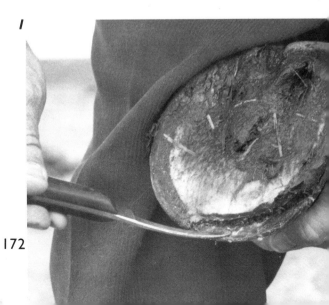

weight of the horse. Subsequently, small stones or dirt pack in and enlarge the space. Occasionally abscesses develop which further complicate the picture (see page 154).

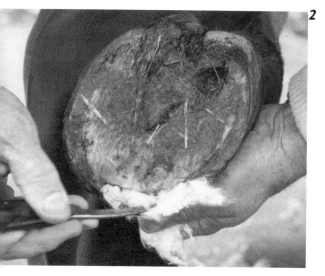

Symptoms
The first sign is usually lameness. Examination of the foot will reveal a dead space filled with debris between the sole and the wall.

Treatment
Remove all dirt and grit and hollow out the seedy toe to its full extent. Then clip and dress the foot. This is a job for your veterinary surgeon or blacksmith.

Pack the cavity with tar and tow or with cotton wool soaked in an oily suspension of antibiotic (*photo 2*), and shoe with a broad-webbed shoe with the web covering the packed cavity.

Some veterinary surgeons recommend cutting away the outer wall of the cavity; others, blistering the coronet to stimulate the growth of new horn. In my opinion neither of these is necessary, provided the foot is subsequently carefully looked after and shod regularly.

98
Thrush

Thrush is a degenerative condition of the frog characterised by a foul smelling discharge (*photo 1*).

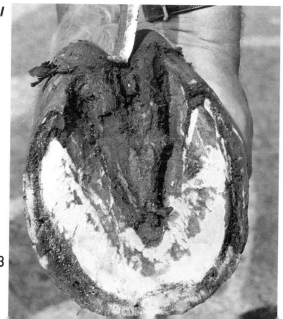

Cause
The predisposing causes are unhygienic conditions and bad management — filthy loose boxes and lack of frog pressure resulting from bad shoeing or poor foot trimming. The frog becomes under-run and bacteria start to multiply; the chief germ has a rather complicated name — *Spherophorus necrophorus*.

Symptoms
The under-run area exudes a black or grey

173

foul-smelling discharge (*photo 2*).

In advanced cases the horse is acutely lame, and the symptoms are identical to those found in the case of a picked-up nail and are caused by the same thing, that is, pressure of the pus on the underlying sensitive laminae.

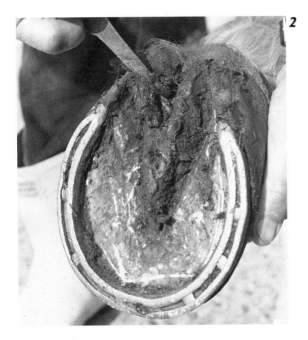

2

Treatment
First of all remove the predisposing causes.

Using a sharp foot knife and scalpel expose all the under-run tissue. If lameness is present, this is a job for the veterinary surgeon.

Wash with soap-flakes and warm water containing a non-irritant antiseptic. Dry thoroughly and spray with a powerful broad-spectrum antibiotic and repeat the spraying once or twice daily until all evidence of discharge has disappeared.

Unfortunately the aerosols containing gentian violet are being taken off the market because the gentian violet is thought to be carcinogenic. However, a suitable substitute will no doubt soon be devised.

If thrush occurs in the summer and the horse is at grass, paint the apparently cured frog with stockholm tar. This will keep the flies away and prevent another flare up of infection.

Prevention
Regular foot inspection and regular shoeing or foot trimming by a competent blacksmith, with the accent on developing and maintaining frog pressure.

99
Canker

Canker can probably be best described as a moist eczema of the sole or frog or more usually both.

Cause
The specific cause is unknown but the predisposing causes are similar to those described for thrush, especially the filthy, unhygienic stable conditions.

Canker used to be fairly common in heavy work horses tied in stables with their hind feet constantly in urine and faeces soaked bedding. Fortunately, with modern loose boxes the

condition is not often encountered.

Symptoms
The sole or frog surface or part of it is covered by a thin scab underneath which is a necrotic or dead moist layer, almost cheeselike, with a peculiar characteristic smell.

Treatment
Certainly a job for a veterinary surgeon. He may or may not anaesthetise the horse but he will surgically remove all the abnormal layer and will apply antibiotic, antiseptic or caustic dressings under pressure.

APPENDIX *Common substances and plants poisonous to horses with any known antidotes*

Substance or Plant	Chief Source	Main Symptoms	Antidote
Lead	Paint or paint-impregnated felt.	Blindness, hyperexcitability, staggering.	Epsom salts given in solution with warm water as a drench or by stomach tube. Epsom salts — magnesium sulphate — makes the insoluble lead salts soluble so that they can be absorbed.
Creosote (Phenol)	Freshly painted boxes or fences or open tins. Creosote applied as a cure for ringworm or lice.	Slobbering, shock, subnormal temperature; rapid pulse; vile-smelling breath; burns in mouth; completely off food and constipated.	Epsom salts given in solution with warm water as a drench or by stomach tube.
Privet	Certain hedges	Horse dies if it eats privet.	No known antidote. Never graze near privet.
Yew	Branches or leaves from yew trees. Usually grown in gardens or parks.	Suddenly fatal.	No known antidote. Never graze near yew trees.
Ragwort	Hay containing the weed.	The horse loses condition. It goes off food and is constipated. The membranes of the mouth and eye become jaundiced because the ragwort damages the liver. The horse starts to stagger sleepily and death soon follows. According to the amount eaten the horse can live for one or more weeks after symptoms start.	Make sure there is no ragwort in the hay because there is no known antidote. The best idea is to kill the ragwort at the bud stage by spraying it early in July. However, if the horse is suspected of having eaten ragwort, a purgative given immediately may prevent the onset of symptoms.
Foxglove	Rough meadow hay.	Death occurs within a few hours if even a small quantity is eaten.	No specific antidote, so make sure there is no foxglove in your hay. Walk the grazing carefully in the early spring and spray any foxglove found.
Deadly nightshade	Certain pastures but rarely in hay.	Fortunately horses will only eat deadly nightshade if virtually starving.	No antidote in horses, so it is well to avoid winter grazing where this plant is growing. Also spray against it in the early spring.
Bracken	Bracken plants especially during a dry season.	Symptoms appear a month or two after first eating the plant. There is a general loss of condition followed by an unsteady gait. Later the horse goes off its food; it shows nervous spasms before death. There is no fever, the patient's temperature remaining normal.	No satisfactory antidote. Avoid use of green bracken as bedding and provide no access to bracken, especially during the winter grazing.

Horse suffering from bracken poisoning (see Appendix)

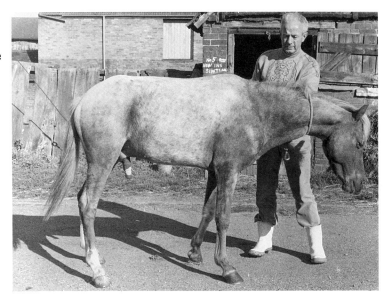

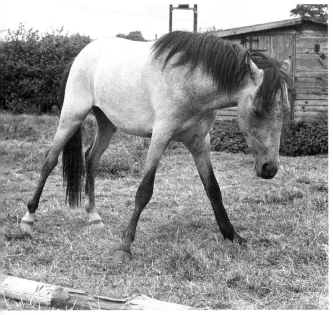

Lead poisoning. The horse is blind and staggering (see Appendix)

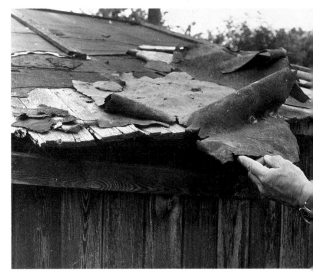

The source of the lead — chewed felt impregnated with lead paint

Index

*For a free illustrated book list containing details of other books by
Eddie Straiton, ring (0473) 241122 or write*

**Farming Press Books
Wharfedale Road, Ipswich IP1 4LG, United Kingdom**

m